Medical Terminology

An Easy and Practical Guide to Better Understand, Pronounce, and Memorize Terms

Nathan Orwell

Table of Contents

INTRODUCTION

"The chapter you're learning today is going to save someone's life tomorrow. Pay attention."

– Khangal Weheartit

Millions of medical students out there struggle to cope with the overwhelming demands of how much they need to learn and memorize as they are exposed to many terminologies. They battle with the expectation always to be ready to remember medical terms when needed, seeing the sensitivity of their profession and how human lives depend on their functionality. Imagine a medical doctor is to clerk a patient but cannot quickly and freely recall terms to diagnose a patient according to what they present. Serious issues can emanate from getting stuck on terminologies, hence the need for medical students to know medical terminologies and also learn how best to easily memorize them to be effective in the course of their practice.

Because of that, this book is purposed to help you assimilate your inevitable medical terms with ease. Moreover, it also provides some fantastic tips to enhance your learning and study culture. So, sit back, relax, and enjoy the book as you read what interests you.

What you must know is that there are thousands of medical terms, and remembering them might prove difficult. However, attempting to remember them is a form of brain exercise. Some people think that one of the reasons we cannot remember the names of people we meet is because we have not paid attention to them in the first place. Pressure, stress, and anxiety can get in the way of the attention needed for memorizing. The number one reason you want to be relaxed when you learn medical terminology is to train yourself to be relaxed when trying to recall the words in normal conversation. It is a terrible experience to forget a known word due to tenseness or a clouded mind. I am sure you are encouraged to explore the relevant tips to learn and memorize your medical tips.

Additionally, this book contains an education on medical terms based on body systems, which will significantly enhance your understanding as you study; these terms are also arranged in alphabetical order for easy comprehension and usage.

CHAPTER 1
Basic Problems in Learning and Memorizing Medical Terminologies

Good memory is a potent quality in everyone's life, especially for students and professionals in different fields. The more improved your memory is, the better your chances to succeed in your profession. As a medical student or expert, think of how wonderful it would be to remember terminologies taught in the class and recall them efficiently in the course of examinations or your practice. Assertiveness is Important not only in memorizing but also in retaining the particular words and pronunciation used. At times, emergencies occur, and you're expected to give quality care amidst the heat of that moment.

A doctor or a nurse is always saddled with assessing, diagnosing, and treating patients without referring to the book when duty calls, just like a pharmacist with his drugs prescriptions; he must use these terms whenever required.

Making The Best Use of Your Memory

Now that you understand the importance of a good memory, you need to master your thinking faculty. To reach the zenith of your memory usage, there are some fundamental things you need to understand to eliminate the initial problem of assimilation and relating with medical terms.

Enhancing Tool for Memory

Do you remember when you checked your entrance examination result into college, met your spouse for the first time, or won a competition? Of course, I am sure you remember that memorable day in its full detail. It should amaze you that without taking classes on "memory techniques," you could recall events that happened in the past. In contrast, if you were asked about the time you put a call through to a fellow last week Monday, your mind would go blank. It will interest you to know that factors, both situational and natural, affect our effectiveness in remembering things. There are two principal components of memory, which are "record" and "recall." When new information is safely stored in the brain, we say it has been recorded. The recorded information requires to be ***recalled*** before we can say that we have ***memorized*** that information. Stored information that cannot be recalled or brought back for use is a waste.

There are some natural factors helpful in converting any information into memory, and they can be summarized in the following order:

- Attention
- Interest
- Emotions

Attention

Scientists have discovered that attention significantly helps the brain in saving new information. Attention is the ability to focus on a task of choice. The brain works on or processes only that task and ignores the rest of the stimuli. Attention is described as a fuss or point of concern, and we avert distraction by focusing. For instance, when in a noisy room, we find it hard to comprehend what a person is saying to us. However, when we focus and carefully select our perception, we discover that it becomes easier to catch the person's voice talking to us. That is achieved by focalizing on one sound and ignoring or neglecting all other sounds.

Series of experiments have revealed that a mere repetition of a task without paying attention fails to create any new neural circuits in the brain, i.e., making repetitions for the sake of repetition will not be of any benefit to you. Some studies by researchers focusing on “memory” have shown that close attention must be given to information when forming long-term memories.

So, “attention” operates as a gate that opens and gives access to more neural information to be digested. It is, therefore, safe to say that without attention, all the information taken in by our senses — what we hear, feel, see, taste, and smell — are technically not registered in our minds.

As humans, our mind is programmed to focus our attention on what we see as "real." So, whatever information we ignore or neglect, despite its importance, seems to fade into insignificance.

Therefore, we must always incline our ears to relevant things so that they can stay in our memory for a long time. We need to pay attention to details.

Interest

Your interest in a particular piece of information precedes and plays a vital role in shaping what you pay attention to when you want to learn and remember something for a more extended period.

Let us check this scenario…

John is all set to go out and play football with his friends when his mom summons him and tells him that he is to run some errands for her at the market. She tells him all she wants him to get for her at the market, but John is not happy about the errand because of the wrong timing. He desperately wants to be on the football pitch with his friends. He listens to his mom with a lackadaisical attitude and heads for the market after. Just as he arrives at the market, it becomes challenging for him to recall what she told him to get.

That happened because John was disinterested in everything his mum told him; that explains why he could not recall everything said to him. That is precisely what the majority of us go through in our daily activities. Most students find it hard to recollect all the things taught to them daily. Of course, that is all because of a lack of interest, but that cannot be your case if you have passion for your course of study.

On the other hand, you can easily maintain your attention to things you are interested in. For example, when last were you distracted by thoughts of your homework or forthcoming exams while watching your favorite movie, game, or TV series? Most people would say, “never.” You could concentrate and pay full attention to a 90-minute football game because you were interested in the game; you gave it your undivided attention. So, when you are about to read, make sure you are in for it. Whatever perception your mind gives it will determine your concentration. Thus, attention is significant whether the information to be memorized is simple or not.

Furthermore, any information that interests you are stored automatically as short-term or long-term memory, depending on your level of interest and emotions attached to the information or event. Also, one crucial thing you must know about interest is that you can generate it.

Emotions

Your emotions play a key role if you would maintain your interest in anything.

For example, as a medical student or expert, you will agree with me that you study voraciously because of the demands of your chosen discipline. Most importantly, you study because of your interest in seeing human bodies recover from illnesses by your knowledge and experience — the passion might not be there if it were another course like law. Even when you encounter difficulties, your love for the discipline of medicine will push you through; hence, our emotions play an essential role in maintaining our interest in something and, in this case, "medical terminologies."

As discussed above, if you do not pay attention, the information will not register inside your brain. We, therefore, can say that attention is equated to a Mental Muscle which can be trained to become stronger and sharper. Nonetheless, you have to desire to work on it.

Quick Exercise 1

1. The 3 natural factors useful in Converting information to memory are ____________, _________, & ____________.

2. The recorded information requires to be __________ before we can say that we have memorized that information.

Easy Ways to Absorb, Retain, And Recall Medical Terminologies

So, you have thought or said, "Medical terminologies are difficult to memorize. How do I master this volume of words?"

Sit back and relax; there is a solution for you.

If you need to memorize difficult, unfamiliar words or names, it would be best to learn an effective method called the Personal Nick Name method. Remember, the Periodic Table and its elements, how you were able to memorize at least the first 20 elements? You either made the first letters of each element into sentences or converted the whole table into a familiar song.

Personal Nick Name (Pnn) Method

When we listen to a complex or long name, we often provide a short (nick) name that simplifies its pronunciation. Also, the new or challenging words we hear should give us instincts to pronounce them slowly or look for a related image already stored in our memory. Then, we can use that similar word as a nickname for the new word.

This proven method of giving a nickname to a new word is known as Personal Nick Name (PNN) method. It can be a singular word or be formed with many words.

Give It a Nickname

For instance, if you want to visualize the name of a body part, such as the Pancreas, it may be challenging at first, especially if you are in the medical field. However, through the PNN system, when we pronounce Pancreas slowly as PAN - K - EARS, we can find some familiar words such as the following:

- Pan
- Pan + Ears

You may also subconsciously imagine some other words. People use different nicknames for different terms; reason for the name, personal nickname method, as it is not fixed and depends on one's imagination and earlier vocabulary.

Now, a word like “Pancreas,” which was earlier difficult for you to visualize, will have a clear image in your mind. Thus, the PNN method is helpful for recalling abstract terms, technical words, scientific jargons, general names, and registers. You do not have to use familiar words to label PNN; other related sounds or pictorial representations will do.

You can take a word, think of any similar knowledge you have on it, and then visualize an image corresponding to both word and the knowledge.

The use of PNN makes it possible to convert any abstract word, phrase, medical and technical terms or complex words into images. It would be easy for you to relate to such information.

A MYTH: People memorize faster when they take pictures of words with their minds and associate with them.

If that were an effective way of learning things, our minds would be clustered with many pictures, confusing and disorienting us.

THE TRUTH: Our brains have a restricted capacity for words but a boundless ability for images or pictures.

Memorizing Medical Terms

This method can be used to learn medical terminologies. For instance, a medical student, who has to memorize the names of various bones in the human body, could find it hard to remember the terms of the wrist bones, i.e., Lunate, Triquetrum, Trapezium, Trapezoid, Hamate, Scaphoid, Pisiform, and Capitate. However, by using the PNN method, one can convert difficult names of bones into simple pictures.

Name of the Bones	**Nicknames (PNN)**
Femur	Fair + more
Phalanges	Far + Ages
Capitate	Cap + it + ate
Hamate	Ham + ate

Quick Exercise 2

1. PNN means ____________________.

2. Give these words PNNs: Scapula, Stomach, Nodular, Ventricle.

3. The brain has a limited capacity for words. True or False?

CHAPTER 2
Ways Of Selecting the Words to Learn

Studying comes with memorizing and, certain variables need to be considered when studying. When you have a strategic way of choosing the words to learn, it becomes easier to flow with them. There are four guidelines that you can use:

Know Why You Study

You know why you eat or sleep. It is so you can be healthy and alert always. The same principle goes for life, and there should be an endpoint as to why you do whatever you do, studying inclusive. You can score yourself based on these questions:

Why am I in Med school?

If you do not know why you are aspiring to be a Doctor or why you are in Med school, you may as well be confused as to why you need to study terminologies.

Maybe, you are following your Parents' or godfather's footsteps, and you do not have that interest at heart; to become a medical practitioner, so much is expected of you, and you are not ready to disappoint people. You have not had a reason to put on a Lab coat or read this book. There are two options here for you: Find a motivation to become a Medical Doctor or Quit. You do not have to subject yourself to unnecessary punishment. You can choose to be a lifesaver or any other esteemed Profession. It is your choice to make. Now, suppose you have got your answer, and it is bending towards the side of continuing this book. In that case, you must apply the same principle to knowing these terminologies. To examine and understand the meaning of words, you first have to ensure they are words that you need to memorize at the moment. There are some words you do not need to engage yourself in learning at the moment. You should not have a test in Anatomy and decide to know all the names of a Chinese Football club's players.

What difference does it make?

Ask yourself what difference it makes if you are not a Doctor but an Astronaut, Engineer, Lawyer, or Teacher. If it makes a difference to you, that is, if you see a reason why you should not be in any of the other professions other than what you are studying, learning your terminologies or not should also make a difference to you. Do not take the comparison literally; every profession is unique. You should focus on the message of the Illustration. You know the difference between getting your snow coat ready for winter and just purchasing the coat when winter comes. Going out on your first date with that person you so much admire, would you leave your hair unkempt? You'd get a haircut or straighten them out if need be, so you look perfect for the moment. Learning your terminologies should be treated just like that. Asking yourself the difference between studying these words and not, you should know why you study. Would you want to be a rusty professional or one that is confident in himself when diagnosing, treating, and educating patients? What difference does it make?

Can I do this?

The last question you should ask yourself in this guideline is if you can study or not. This question would pop up anytime you are in the problematic zone of memorizing words. As important as the question is, your response is the ultimate. Will like you to think of it as if you're getting admitted into medical school to learn the basics of advanced terminologies. It is that simple. You will know how you can stay put amidst the turbulence of learning words as you continue reading. If you think you can, then yes! You can, and if you believe otherwise, you have the power to change that decision.

Take Your Time to Isolate Categories

Do not just rush into learning all the terminologies simultaneously; you will work yourself out. You might want to use a month on each type of term based on your preference. For instance, you could focus on body parts or diseases, bearing in mind that diseases come with treatment. You might exclude the treatment categories and learn more about them over the long run.

There are a few questions you may want to ask yourself, such as, "Why is it that I want to know this particular word?" "Do I need the word for a particular seminar or presentation?" "Am I learning it to understand a book I am currently reading?" Those are all important questions. Here are some groupings that could help in isolating categories:

Eponyms

These are terminologies named after the person who discovered that disease or body part. Addison's disease, Maslow's hierarchy of needs, Cushing syndrome are all examples of Eponyms.

Homonyms

These are terminologies that sound alike but have entirely different meanings. Examples:

Cholic: An acid//Colic: Severe abdominal pain.

Exemia: loss of fluids (from vessels)//Eczema: Dermatitis.

Ilium: A pubic bone//Ileum: A part of the intestine.

Palpation: A type of examination//Palpitation: Rapid heartbeat.

You might also ask if the word is a synonym. Synonyms are words that have different spellings and pronunciations but likely meanings.

Drug/Medication

Narcotic/Opiate

Sedative/Tranquilizer

Organs/Visceral

It would be best if you developed an eagerness always to study synonyms.

Consider How the Medical Term Will Be in A Sentence

If you cannot immediately think of how it is used, search for an example using a medical dictionary or print resource. It is always worth learning medical terms, even if you do not have a feel for how you might use them. When working to overcome procrastination, you will feel that much more progress has been gained by learning terms that can be put into practice with more imminence. You can call your friends, family, or colleagues by those terms ensuring they are okay with it or use those words while discussing with them. Another idea is to teach them what you have learned. Telling others about what you know makes you recall more about it.

Motivate Yourself

This is done when you think about what you could achieve by having this new word firmly entrenched in your mind. That is a beautiful way to find the drive for learning.

Everyone wants a good memory, but it has to be built and improved over time. Moreover, our desire plays a significant role in concentrating on what we seek to learn and remember. So, the key to placing something is paying close attention to the subject or, in this context, terminology, and not just a mere glancing through. Motivating yourself will excite you, have a reward in mind for every landmark you make memorizing these words. You can decide to go to the mall with your friends after you have learned about 50 Medical Acronyms.

Concentration Enhancement

Meditation is one of such important practices that you have to learn to achieve your set aim. A part of the human brain called the "thalamus" serves as a channel to the sensory information: smell, touch, and sound into the brain. When this information enters the brain, you can claim to be "aware" of it. So, one of the advantages of the practice of meditation is that it finds a way to disallow the influence of other forms of information that might disturb you.

What then is this meditation?

When we enable our mind by focusing our thoughts in a particular direction, that practice is described as "meditation." Ideas are naturally created in our minds; hence, the act of meditating is not just to concentrate on a point or stop all views; however, many times, a whole lot of ideas enter our minds such that we might find it hard to think and focus on what we plan to study or learn. One of the benefits of practicing meditation is the relaxation achieved by sieving and reducing the series of reviews on the mind. Another benefit is the correction and cleansing of wasteful and negative thoughts for the positive ones, hence the need to be deliberate with the practice.

This practice of meditation can be described and split into three levels which are;

1. Self-reflection
2. Mind relaxing
3. Mind recharging

Let us expound on the above-listed steps or levels in the practice of meditation:

Self-reflection

People are often found spending time; watching, viewing, and thinking about others. Many times, we are discovered judging ourselves based on a person's opinions about us; nonetheless, what happens when we meditate is that while we comfortably have our sit, we refuse to think about another person's opinions about us. Instead, we start to observe ourselves, and it appears to be an act of self-examination and brooding.

Mind relaxing

Having observed the ideas, you need to direct the flow of thoughts based on the proper knowledge. It is done just like a disconnected observer; hence, you pay attention to the thoughts you are creating and associate them accordingly with the ones you ought to make at that very moment. So, your responsibility is to get rid of the negative or waste thoughts, whether concerning others or even yourself; hence, relaxing your mind by reducing the encumbrance. Be sure to choose what ideas you take on carefully.

Mind recharging

At this juncture, you then have to make a deliberate effort towards making positive thoughts and to ensure that you remain in that consciousness, having ascertained the right mindfulness about yourself, including your inner strength. Do not forget the fact that you can make your choice in creating powerful and positive thoughts. By this, you get to feel good and energized. So, when we meditate, we also visualize the thoughts made and ensure to remain in mindedness.

Quick Exercise 3

1. The part of the brain that serves as a channel to the sensory information: smell, touch, and sound is the ___________?

2. Through meditation, we can sieve and reduce the series of thoughts in our minds. True or False?

3. What three essential questions should you ask yourself to know why you study?

CHAPTER 3
Introduction To Word Parts and Construction

Sequel to the preceding chapter that focused on "the basic problems in learning and memorizing medical terminologies," we succeeded in explaining the practical ways by which you can easily assimilate the volume of things to learn, medical words, and the seemingly difficult words procedures that are relevant to your profession.

Consequently, this chapter seeks to allay your fears regarding how to intelligently use terminologies from the vast medical vocabulary when needed without any qualms. In furtherance to the methods explained in the earlier chapter, there is yet another more relevant one that facilitates an easy recall of medical terminologies. To your utmost advantage, it would not just enhance your ability to recall because, as you must have learned in the previous chapter, the mind quickly becomes full of words. At the same time, it remains ready to receive information in a pictorial format. So, this chapter will familiarize you with how to have your way around medical words, dissect them, and how to determine the meaning of these terms by using word roots, prefixes, suffixes, and word combinations. It will also enhance your informed guessing skill when faced with some strange terms.

Very importantly, if you can master the building blocks or word parts that make up every medical term by carefully analyzing and identifying the word roots, prefixes, suffixes, and word combinations, you have all it takes to be confident as a medical professional with the use medical terminologies that have become your daily mode of interaction in the medical world.

Word parts: This refers to the various entities that make up medical terminologies. They are broken into word roots, prefixes, suffixes, and word combinations. A good understanding of interpreting each part will help simplify the mountain of seeming complex medical terminologies.

Word root(s): They are the primary or fundamental part or element of all medical terminologies. They tell us the meaning, focus, or direction of the word. It can either be one or more in every medical term and is fondly called "a root," but it should be noted that it can stand alone or be combined with other elements to develop another medical word with a different meaning.

For instance, in the English language, we can also have word roots and identify them for easy comprehension.

The word "teach" is the root word for **teach**er, **teach**es, **teach**ing.

The word "drive" is the root word for **driv**er, **driv**ing, **drive**s.

The word "beauty" is the root word for **beaut**iful.

It, therefore, suggests that if I can separate the word parts or elements into their components, which are; word roots, prefixes, suffixes, and word combinations. It thus means that I can understand what the medical word or terminology is about by simply identifying the word root(s).

Another instance:

Stand Alone	**As part of a word**
Sperm	**Sperm**icide (what kills

	sperm)
Insect	**Insect**icide (what kills insects)
Glucose	**Glyco**suria (Glucose in the urine)
Protein	**Protein**uria (Protein in the urine)

Commonly, medical terminologies are derived from Greek and Latin words.

Dentist - the root word here is the word "dent," used for a tooth.

Dermatologist - the root word here is the word “dermat,” used for the skin.

Pancreatitis - the root word here is the word “pancreat,” used for the pancreas.

Further to what has been said about “word root(s),” it should be noted that these words are either from Greek or Latin languages. That could be the reason why we can have two words say similar things.

For instance:

Greek	Latin	Meaning
Derm	Cutane	Skin
Nephr	Ren	Kidney

Fundamentally, you will often see Greek word roots being used to develop or build words addressing diagnosis, diseases, treatments, and conditions whereas, Latin words are often used to describe body structures or anatomy.

Combining form: The best thing to do in learning a word root is to learn its **combining vowel** alongside. When a word root and its vowel are put together, it is called "**combining form**."

Let us quickly learn what a combining vowel is to enhance our knowledge of "combining words."

Combining vowels is often "**O**," and it's used only if the suffix attached to the word root doesn't start with a vowel but consonant.

For instance:

The word "**arthritis**" can be broken down into "**arthr**" and "**itis**," where the word "**itis**" is the suffix, and "**arthr**" remains the word root. That is because the suffix started with a vowel "**Itis**"; hence, no **combining vowel** would be added.

On the contrary, let us observe an instance where a combining vowel is used. Of course, the criteria would be that the suffix joining the word root must start with a consonant letter to leave room for the combining vowel.

For instance:

Hematology can be broken into; hemat – **o** – logy. Here, the word root is "**hemat**," "**logy**," is the suffix, while "**o**" is the combining vowel. Observe the rule again; the combining vowel was used simply because the suffix "**logy**" starts with the letter "**l**ogy," a consonant. In this case, it is used to combine a word root and a suffix.

In addition, a "**combining vowel,**" majorly "O," can be used to join two-word roots.

Osteoarthritis – there are two-word roots here to be identified: "**Oste**," referring to the bone, and the word "**arthr**," referring to joint. Also, the suffix here is the word “**itis**,” and the letter “**O**” that comes in-between “oste” and “arthr” is the combining vowel. It should be noted that the suffix, which is the word “it is,” implies an inflammation. So, putting this together, the word “osteoarthritis” would mean an inflammation of the bone and joint.

So, a “combining form” is a term used to describe the name of a word root with a combining vowel.

Examples

Aden/o, Athr/o, Hemat/o, Arter/o, Neur/o, Lymph/o, Cardi/o, Encephal/o, and Therm/o

Now, let us split it.

Word Root	**Vowel**	**Combining From**	**Meaning**
Aden/	O	Aden/o	It refers to the Gland.
Arthr/	O	Arthr/o	It refers to the joint.

Articul/		Articul/o	
Hemat/	O	Hemat/o	It refers to the blood.
Neur/	O	Neur/o	It refers to the Nerves.
Lymph/	O	Lymph/o	It refers to the Lymph.
Cardi/	O	Cardi/o	It refers to the Heart.
Encephal/	O	Encephal/o	It refers to the brain.
Erythr/	O	Erythr/o	It refers to a red color.

Hepat/	O	Hepat/o	It refers to the Liver.
Nephr/	O	Nephr/o	It refers to the Kidney.
Arteri/ Arter/	O O	Arteri/o Arter/o	They both refer to the **artery**.
Ather/	O	Arther/o	It refers to a plaque or fat.
Carcin/	O	Carcin/o	It relates to cancer.
Bronch/	O	Bronch/o	It refers to the bronchus.

Chol/	E	Chol/e	It deals with the Bile.
Cholecyst	O	Cholecyst/o	It relates to the gall bladder.
Enter/	O	Enter/o	It refers to the intestine.
Cyt/	O	Cyt/o	It refers to the cells.
Galact/	O	Galact/o	It refers to milk.
Glyc/	O	Glyc/o	It refers to sugar.
Gynec/	O	Gynec/o	It refers to

			females.
Hemat/ Hem/	O	Hemat/o Hem/o	It has to do with the blood.
Hyster/	O	Hyster/o	It refers to the Uterus.
Latr/	O	Latr/o	It refers to a treatment.
Leuk/	O	Leuk/o	It refers to a white color.
Men/	O	Men/o	It refers to menses or mensuration in females.

My/	O	My/o	It refers to the muscles.
Myel/	O	Myel/o	It refers to the bone marrow or spinal cord.
Necr/	O	Necr/o	It refers to death.
Nat/	O	Nat/o	It refers to birth.
Pharmac/	O	Pharmac/o	It deals with drugs.
Phleb/	O	Phleb/o	It deals with the veins.

Phren/	O	Phren/o	It deals with the diaphragm.
Pleur/	O	Pleur/o	It deals with the pleura or ribs.
Pneum/ Pulmon/	A or O O	Pneum/a or /o Pulmon/o	It deals with the lungs.
Proct/	O	Proct/o	It refers to the rectum or anus.
Py/	O	Py/o	It deals with the pus.

Sept/	O	Sept/o	It refers to an infection.
Testicul/	O	Testicul/o	It refers to the testis.
Thorac/	O	Thorac/o	It refers to the chest.
Thyr/	O	Thyr/o	It refers to the thyroid gland.
Tranche/	O	Tranche/o	It refers to the trachea.
Thym/	O	Thym/o	It refers to the thymus.

Recall that the combining vowel that makes up the combining form (Word roots + combining vowel) is only relevant if the suffix or the word root that comes after it starts with a consonant letter.

Take Neur**itis,** for instance. The combining vowel "O" is not used because our suffix starts with a vowel.

Suffix(es): It is a part of the word root that can tell us more about the word root. When you hear about the word "suffix," what ought to first come to your mind is its position at the end of word root in many cases. It can also come after a prefix. Secondly, you must have questions running through your mind. That is because a suffix will inform you of the problem, procedure, disease, and condition.

For instance:

Suffixes	**Meaning**
-itis	Inflammation.
-ectomy	Removal, excision.

-megaly	Enlargement.
-oma	Tumor.
-ia, -osis, -ism	Condition.
-ar, -ic, -um, -tic, -ous	Relating to, as regards.
-logy	Study.
-meter	Measurement.
-therapy	Treatment.
-algia	Pain.
-stomy	New opening.

-phasia	Speaking.
-pathy	Disease.
-emia	Condition of blood.
-gram	A record or image.
-iatry	Specialty.
-logist	Someone who studies.
-philia	Affinity for loving.
-scope	An instrument used to view something.
-drome	When something is running.
-malacia	Refers to a softening.

-opsy	To view or examine.
-oxia	A condition concerning Oxygen.
-phagia	A condition that deals with **eating or swallowing**.
-physis, -plasia	It deals with **growth**.
-plegia	It deals with **paralysis**.
-stasis	It deals with standing still.
-astenia	It deals with weakness.
-artresia	It deals with a closure or the absence of a normal body opening.

-cele	It refers to swelling, hernia, or protrusion.
-penia	It deals with a deficiency or an abnormality reduction in the number.
-phobia	It refers to a fear of something.
-rrhagia, -rrhea	It is used for an abnormal discharge.
-sclerosis	It refers to a condition of hardening.
-spasm	It refers to what is sudden or involuntary.
-practic	It deals with practice.
-cyte	It refers to cells.
-uria	It deals with urine.

Suffixes Concerning Procedures and Treatments

Suffixes	Meaning
-pexy	It means a surgical fixation or a suspension.
-phylaxis	It means protection.
-plasty	It is used for surgical repair.
-rrhaphy	It is the term used for suturing.
-scopy	The process of viewing.
-stomy	It refers to the surgical creation of an opening.
-tome	It refers to a cutting instrument.
-tomy	It refers to an incision or a cutting.
-tripsy	It refers to a surgical

	crushing.
-ion	It refers to a process.
-lysis	It refers to when something is loosened or dissolved.
-desis	It refers to binding together.
-centesis	It means to puncture

Quick Exercise 4

1. Word parts can contain word roots, prefixes, suffixes and ___________.

2. It is possible to have 2-word roots in a word part. True or False?

3. Give three examples of more than one-word root in a medical word part.

4. Separate the following into word roots, combining vowels and suffixes: Menopause, Hemorrhagic, Cholelithiasis, Homeopathy.

Prefixes

Prefix(es): A prefix contrary to a suffix is a word element that precedes a word root. It can also be added directly in front of a suffix. It Is important to bear in mind that hundreds into thousands of prefixes give direction to the word roots; hence, it is essential to understand them as it helps you identify diseases and everything concerning medicine and its treatments. It would interest you to know that prefixes in medical terminologies can be classified into various forms of their usages. The following are the categories of their classification;

- Prefixes according to **Numbers**
- Prefixes according to **Colors**
- Prefixes according to **Negativity**
- Prefixes according to **Direction**
- Prefixes according to **Degree**
- Prefixes according to **Size and Comparison**
- Prefixes according to **Time**
- Prefixes according to **Position/Location**
- Prefixes according to **Special qualities**

Prefixes according to **Numbers**

Prefix	**Meaning**	**Usage**
Prim/i-	It refers to what comes "first."	Primigravida refers to a first birth
Mon/o-	It refers to what is "one."	Monocular refers to one or a singular eyepiece.
Uni-	It refers to what is "one."	Union refers to the oneness.
Hemi-	It refers to what is "half or one-sided."	Hemisphere refers to one half of a round structure.
Semi-	It refers to what is "half or partial."	Semipermeable refers to what is partially capable of allowing penetration.
Bi-	It refers to what is "two or twice."	Binary refers to what has two parts to it.
Di-	It refers to what is "two or twice."	Diatomic refers to what has two atoms.

Dipl/o	It refers to what is "double."	Diplococci refers to a round-shaped bacteria which grows in groups of two.
Tri-	It refers to what is "three or thrice."	Tricuspid refers to when something has three cusps or points.
Quadr/i-	It refers to what is "four."	Quadruplet indicates four babies that were born together.
Tetra-	It refers to what is "four."	Tetralogy refers to a group of four.
Multi-	It refers to what is "many."	Multicellular refers to many cells.
Poly-	It refers to what is "many or much."	Polymorphous refers to what has many forms.

Prefixes according to **Colors**

Prefix	**Meaning**	**Usage**
Cyan/o-	The word **cyan** deals with a blue color.	The word **cyanosis** speaks of a bluish discoloration found on the skin because of a lack of oxygen.
Erythr/o-	The word **erythr** deals with a red color.	The word **erythrocyte** describes a red blood cell.
Leuk/o-	The word **leuk** deals with the white color.	The word **leukocyte** describes a white blood cell. We can as well have the word **leukemia** which refers to cancer of white blood cells.
Melan/o	The word **melan** deals with black or dark color.	The word **melanin** describes a pigment found in the body responsible for the dark or black color of

		the hair and skin.
Xanth/o	The word **xanth** deals with a yellow color.	The word **xanthoma** describes a yellow cancerous growth found on the skin.

Prefixes according to **Negativity**

Prefix	**Meaning**	**Usage**
a-, an-	They are words used as; **not, lack of something, without, and absence.**	The word **anhydrous** is a word that describes a deficiency or absence of water.
Anti-	This word means **against.**	The word **antiseptic** is a word that describes an agent or material that prevents infection.
Contra-	It is the word that means; against, opposite, opposed.	The word **contraindicated** is a word used to describe what opposes the

		recommendations.
De-	It is a word that means; down, without, removal, loss.	The word **decalcify** means to remove calcium from something.
Dis-	It is a word that means; absence, removal, separation.	The word **dissect** is a word that means to separate tissues.
In-, im-	They are words that mean **not.**	The word **incontinent** is a word that means not able to hold or control a discharge.
Non-	It is a word that means **not.**	The word **noncontributory** is a word that means not significant maybe to a medical diagnosis.
Un-	It is a word that means **not** or	The word **uncoordinated** is a word that means not working together or not

	negation.	coordinated.
Dys-	It is a word that means **Pain.**	The word **dysmenorrhea** is a word that means painful menstruation.
Mal-	It is a word that means **Abnormal** or depicts **Abnormality.**	The word **malformation** is a word that means an abnormal formation.

Prefixes according to **Direction**

Prefix	**Meaning**	**Usage**
Ab-	It is a word that means **away from, take away.**	The word **Abduction** means away from the body.
Ad-	It is a word that means **toward, near.**	The word **Adduction** means towards the body.
Circum-	It is a word that means **around.**	The word **Circumcision** means cutting around the tip of

		the Penis.
Dorsi-/Dorso-	They are words that mean **back** or **posterior**.	The word **Dorsiflexion** means backward flexion.
Flex-	It is a word that means **bend** or **away from**.	The word **Flexion** means the movement of a joint away from the angle between the bones.
Infra-	It is a word that means **below** or **beneath**.	The word **Infratemporal** means below the temporal bone.
Para-	It is a word that means **near** or **beside** or **alongside**.	The word **Paraumbilical** means alongside the umbilicus.
Retro-	It is a word that means **behind** or **backward**.	The word **Retrolingual** means behind the tongue.
Super-	It is a word that means **on top**.	The word **Superiorly** means Organs (or

		structures) on top of the main structure.
Ventro-	It is a word that means **front** or **in front**.	The word **Ventrolateral** means extending from the front and side.

Prefixes according to **Degree**

Prefix	**Usage**	**Meaning**
An-	It is a word that means **not, without, lacking**.	The word **Anovulation** means without ovulation or lacking ovulation.
Brady-	It is a word that means **slow**.	The word **Bradycardia** means slow heart rate.
Hyper-	It is a word that means **high**.	The word **Hyperglycemia**

		means high blood glucose.
Hypo-	It is a word that means **low**.	The word **Hypotension** means low blood pressure.
Mega-	It is a word that means **great or abnormally large**.	The word **Megaloblastic (anemia)** means anemia characterized by very large and abnormal red blood cells.
Oligo-	It is a word that means **few, scanty, small quantity**.	The word **Oligospermia** means scanty urine.
Poly-	It is a word that means **excessive**.	The word **Polyhydramnios** means excessive

		amniotic fluid.
Sub-	It is a word that means below or less than normal.	The word **Subtotal** means less than the total gland or organ as in (thyroidectomy or hysterectomy).
Tachy-	It is a word that means **fast** or **rapid**.	The word **Tachypnea** means rapid respiration.

Prefixes according to Size and Comparison

Prefix	**Usage**	**Meaning**
Ambi- Amphi-/Ampho-	They are words that refer to **both sides, fond of both**.	The word **Ambidextrous** means being able to use both hands equally well The word **Amphophil**

		means a cell that stains both acids and dyes.
Dipl-	It is a word that means **double** or **pairs**.	The word **Diplococcus** means bacteria in pairs.
Macro-	it is a word that means **large, long**.	The word **Macrophages** means large specialized engulfing cells.
Mega-	It is a word that means **great, large**.	The word **Megaloblastic (anemia)** means anemia characterized by very large and abnormal red blood cells.
Micro-	It is a word that	**The word**

	means **small.**	**Microscope** means a device specialized in viewing small organisms.
Semi-	It is a word that means **half**.	The word **Semicanal (of the ear)** means half canal.

Prefixes according to **Time**

Prefix	Usage	Meaning
Ante-/Pre-/ Pro-	These words mean **comes before or before**.	The word **Antepartum** means before childbirth **Preoperatively** means before surgical procedure.

Post-	It refers to **after**.	The word **Postpartum** means after childbirth.
Retro-	It means **back in time**.	**Retrospective data** means medical data and history collected back in time.

Prefixes according to **Position/Location**

Prefixes	**Meaning**	**Usage**
Con-/Co-	These are words that mean **together** or **with**.	The word Convoluted tubules coiled together tubules of the nephron.
Ec-/Ecto-/Extra-/Exo-	These words mean **outside**.	The word **Ectopic Pregnancy** means

		pregnancy occurring outside the uterus. The word **Extracellular** means outside the cell membrane, and the word **Exophthalmos** means the condition where eyeballs protrude outside the eye socket.
Endo-/Intra-	These words refer to **within**.	The word **Endometrium** means the lining within the uterus or inner layer lining the uterus structurally. The word **Intra-abdominal**

		infection refers to the infection affecting the abdominal organs.
Epi-	This word means **upon, over, above**.	The **Epigastric** means the region over/above the stomach.
Eso-	This word means **inward**.	The word **Esotropia** means inward deviation of one or both eyes.
Hypo-	It is a word that means **below**.	The word **Hypodermis** means below the dermis of the skin.
Juxta-	It is a word that means **near**.	The word **Juxtaglomerular** apparatus is a structure located near the glomerulus

		of the kidney.
Peri-	It is a word that means **around**.	The word **Periorbital edema** means swelling around the eyes.
Supra- /Super-	These words mean **above**.	The word **Suprapubic** means above the pubis.

Now, observe that certain prefixes appeared in more than one category; **Semi, Diplo, Poly, Contra, An, and Hypo.** The word root and corresponding suffix will give accurate meaning to the medical term.

Apart from the categories listed above, you should know that certain words do or do not fit into any of these categories. They are referred to as **Prefixes with special qualities** and listed below;

Pseudo, Neo, Pan, Ultra, Meta, Syn, Bio, Necro, Auto, Apo, Eu, and Iso.

Prefixes according to **Special qualities**

Prefixes	Meaning	Usage
Pseudo-	It is a word that means **false**.	The word **Pseudocyst** means false cysts because they do not contain true characteristics of cysts.
Neo-	It is a word that means **new**.	The word **Neonate** refers to a newborn baby.
Pan-	It is a word that means **all**.	The word **Pandemic** means all over the world.
Ultra-	It is a word that means **beyond normal**.	The word **Ultrasound** is imaging that takes pictures of tissues, organs, or other structures beyond what is

		visible.
Meta-	It is a word that means **change**.	The word **Metabolism** means chemical reactions involving a series of events that changes food into energy.
Syn-	It is a word that means **together**.	A word **Syndrome** is a group or collection of many symptoms.
Bio-	It is a word that means **life**.	The word **Biometrics** refers to measurements that identify life characteristics in an individual.
Necro-	It is a word that	The word

	means **death**.	**Necrotizing fasciitis** is the term used to describe a bacterial infection that eats flesh, spreads quickly, and causes death.
Auto-	It is a word that means **self**.	The word **Autonomy** refers to the ability to decide by oneself.
Apo-	It is a word that means **separated, away**.	The word **Apoptosis** means death and separation of cells that occurs as a normal part of an organism's growth and development.

Eu-	It is a word that refers to **normal, genuine**.	The word **Eubacteria** means true bacteria.
Iso-	It is a word that means **uniformity, equality**.	The word **Isotonic solution** refers to a solution that has the same concentration of salt and blood/cells.

Quick Exercise 5

1. Prefixes are also according to categories. List them.
2. Give the categories that the following prefixes belong to; around, large, two, many, all, red, death, away.

CHAPTER 4
Basic Medical Terminologies

As you have earlier learned that Latin words mainly describes body structures or anatomy while Greek words mainly describe diagnoses, diseases, and treatments, we'll examine some basic medical terminologies as they pertain to Anatomy, Medical or Surgical interventions, Diagnostic procedures, Pharmacology, Plural forms of suffixes and word roots in this chapter. These terms may have their origins in ancient Greek and Latin. Note: in this chapter, you will also come across words used in the medical field that do not take their origin from them. Terms that include, Anatomical positions, Acronyms, and Eponyms do not bow to Latin nor Greek.

Anatomy Is Anatomy

Your current year in Med school or how long you have been practicing medicine does not matter; the definition of anatomy remains unchanged. Just like your name is not changing anytime soon unless you decide to start a whole new life, it will be foolish for health professionals to have different ideas of what the human anatomy is about.

Ana- up
Tome- cutting

Anatomy is derived from the **Greek** word **Ana** which means **"up,"** and **tome,** which is to "**cut through**." You can say Human Anatomy is the cutting up of the human body. Of course, it would not just be dissecting the human body for fun but for study, to know more. A refined definition goes, Human anatomy is the study of the structures of the body, and with study comes organizations. Think about it, how inconvenient and unpleasant it would be to cut the liver and the bones simultaneously. That's how the study of anatomy is without first organization; hence, the study of Human Anatomy can be organized into three types.

Regional Anatomy: This is the organization and study of the human body into defined parts; head, neck, upper limb, lower limb, abdomen, thorax, trunk, and pelvis

Systemic Anatomy**:** This is the organization and study of the human body into systems: Integumentary, circulatory, respiratory, lymphatic, reproductive, endocrine, nervous, digestive, skeletal, and urinary.

Microscopic Anatomy: This is the organization and study of the human body, which cannot be seen with the naked eye: cells and tissues.

What then is an Anatomical Position?

A body in Anatomical Position stands upright with arms at each side and palms facing forward. The feet side by side and toes pointed outwards. This is the acceptable default position a body can assume. Other positions discussed below are assumed for examination and treatment purposes.

Medical Terminologies According to Anatomical Positions

Term	Meaning	Type of word	Origin	Meaning	Procedures
Prone	It means when the	Word root	Latin: **Pronus**	Bent forward.	Neurosurgeries, Assessment of the

	person lies horizontally with face and torso facing down.				Dorsal Aspects of the body.
Supine	It means the person lies horizontally with face and torso facing down.	Word root	Latin: **suppinus**	Thrown backward.	General Assessment of the body, Procedures involving lower extremities, Abdominal surgeries

					, Cardiac surgeries .
Semi-Recumbent	It means the person lies with the head and torso at an angle of 45 degrees.	Prefix: Re Word root: Cumbent	Latin: **Re** Latin: **Cumbere**	Backward. To lie down, Recline.	Extubation.
Lateral Recumbent	It means the person lies	Prefix: Lateral Prefix/ Word	Latin: **Lateralis** Latin: **Re,**	Belonging to the side.	Procedures involving the Thorax,

	horizontally with either the left or right side.	root: ReCumbent	**Cumbere**	Backward, Recline.	Kidneys, and Hips.
Knee-chest	This means the person rests on the knee and chest with head turned to a side, the				A lumbar procedure like Lumbar puncture, Rectal examination, Surgeries involving the Genitals.

	elbows and flexed but arms are extended on a horizontal surface.				
Litothomy	This means the person lies horizontally on the back, and the	Word root: Lith Combining vowel: O Suffix: Tomy	Greek: **Lithos** Greek: **Tomo**	Stone Cut	During Childbirth, Gynecological examinations and surgeries, Rectal examination.

	legs flexed at 90degree, hips also flexed.				
Trendelenburg	This means the person lies on the back, knees and legs are flexed, upper body about	Word root	German Surgeon: **Fredrick Trendelenburg**		Surgical procedures involving the Genitourinary and Abdominal organs.

	45 degrees but lower than the rest of the body.				

There are so many Anatomical positions with Latin origin for different purposes. As you get involved more in the practice of medicine, you come across these terms more. Some others are, **Sims position, Low recumbent position, and Knee-elbow positions**

What about Body planes?

Body planes are imaginary planes used to divide the body into sections to describe the locations and directions of the body structures.

Medical Terminologies According to Body Planes

Term	Meaning	Type of	Origin	Meaning

		word		
Sagittal	This means the body is **cut into two halves: forward and backwar d**.	Word root: Sagitt/Suffi x: -al	Latin: **Sagittus**	Arrow (somethi ng that cuts through from front to back).
Coronal	This means the body is **cut into two halves: side to side**.	Word root: Coron/Suffi x: -al	Latin; **Coronal is**	Crown
Median	This means that the	Word root	Latin: **Medus**	Middle

	body is **cut vertically in the middle into equal halves**.			
Transverse	This means that the body is **cut across into top and bottom halves**.	Prefix: Trans Word root: Verse	Latin: **Trans** Latin: **Vertere**	Across To turn
Oblique	This means that the body **is not cut**	Word root	Latin: **Obliquus**	Slanting

	into any of the above planes but cut slant.			

What are Directional terms?

Directional terms are terms that describe the position of structures in relation to other structures in the human body.

Medical Terminologies According to Direction

Term	Meaning	Type of word	Origin	Meaning	Usage
Anterior (Ventral)	This means the structure is situated in front of the	Word root: Ante Suffix: rior	Latin	**In front of, before.**	The thoracic cage is anterior to the Heart.

	determining structure.				
Posterior (Dorsal)	This refers to the structure situated at the back of the determining structure.	Word root: Poste Suffix: rior	Latin: Posterus	**Coming after**.	The Pectoralis Major is posterior to the Breast.
Superior	This refers to the structure situated	Word root: Super Suffix:	Latin: Superus	**That is above**	The eyelids are superior to the

	above or on top of the determining structure.	rior			eyeballs.
Inferior	This refers to the structure situated below the determining structure.	Word root: Infe Suffix: rior	Latin: Inferus	**Below**	The abdomen cavity is inferior to the cranial cavity.
Lateral	This refers to the	Word root:	Latin: Lateralis	**Belonging to the**	The ovaries are

	structure situated to the side of the determining structure.	Later Suffix: al		**side**.	lateral to the Uterus.
Proximal	This refers to the structure situated near the center axis of the determining structur	Word root Suffix: al	Latin: Proximus	**Nearest to**	The fingers are proximal to the wrist.

	e.				
Distal	This refers to the structure situated away from the center axis of the determining structure.	Word root: Dist Suffix: al	Latin: Distare	**To stand away from.**	The fingers are distal to the elbow.
Cephalic	This means that the structure is directed towards	Word root: Cephal Suffix: ic	Greek: Kephale	**Head**	The fetus has a Cephalic presentation.

	the head.				
Caudal	This means that the structur e is directed towards the tail.	Word root: Caud Suffi x: al	Greek: Caudal	**Tail**	Caudal equina is the collectio n of nerves at the tail end of the spinal cord.
Superfi cial	This means the structur e that is towards the body surface or the determi	Word root: Super fic Suffi x: al	Latin: Superfic ialis	**Pertain ing to the surface**	The jugular vein is superfici al to the skin of the neck.

	ning structur e.				
Deep	This means the structur e that is inward and away from the body surface or the determi ning structur e.	Word root			The Endomet rium is deep to the pelvic outlet.

Always remember:

Suffix: **-al means Pertaining to.**

Suffix: **-ic also means Pertaining to.**

Body Cavities

Body cavities are spaces that occupy visceral (internal organs, fluids, connecting structures). The body without the arms and legs (appendages or limbs) is known as the torso or trunk and head. Unlike the limbs, the Trunk and head are not solid-like but contain different structures such as the lubricating fluids, membranes, and organs.

The body cavities are divided into two by direction: The Dorsal cavity and the Ventral Cavity are divided into Structures and Functions:

Cranial Cavity

Spinal Cavity

Thoracic Cavity

Abdominal Cavity

Pelvic Cavity

The Cranial and Spinal Cavities are positioned Dorsally (At the back), while the other three Cavities are positioned Ventrally (At the front).

Medical Terminologies According to Body Cavities

Term	Word type	Origin	Structures
Cranial	Word root: Crani/Suffix: -al	Latin: Cranium Greek: Kranion	**Brain and Meninges.**
Spinal	Word root: Spin/Suffix: -al	Latin: Spinalis	**Spinal column.**
Thoracic Pericardial Pleural	Word root: Thorac/Suffix: -ic Prefix: Peri/Word root: Cardi/Suffix: -al Word root:	Latin: Thoracicus Greek: Peri Greek: Cardion Greek: Pleuron	**Esophagus, trachea, lungs, heart, aorta** **Areas that surrounds the heart** **Ribs** **Heart, great**

Mediastinum	Pleur/Suffix: -al Word root: Media/Word root: Stinum	Latin: Medius Greek: Sternon	**blood vessels, and thymus gland.**
Abdominal	Word root: Abdomin/Suffix: -al	Latin: Abdomin	**Kidneys, Intestines, Liver, Stomach, Spleen, Ureters, Pancreas, Gall bladder.**
Pelvic	Word root: Pelv/Suffix: -ic	Latin: Peluis/Pelvis	**Urinary Bladder, Vagina, Large intestines (part), Uterus,**

			Rectum (part), Prostrate.

Take Note: The Thoracic Cavity is divided into the **Pericardial cavity, Pleural Cavity, and the Mediastinum.**

The Pleural cavity consists of the following:

Visceral Pleural: Serous membrane that is attached directly to the Lungs.

Parietal Pleural: Serous membrane that lines the inner wall of the Chest.

Combining Directional Terms

In your study and practice, you'll come across terms that include 2-word roots. A Combining vowel is used to build those words. Here are some **2-word roots.**

Anteroinferior

Anterolateral

Posteroinferior

Posterolateral

Superolateral

Cephalocaudal

Abdominopelvic

Thoracolumbar

Abdominal Regions and Quadrants

The Abdomen is large and houses many organs; hence, it is divided into four Quadrants and nine Regions to facilitate easy recognition of organs and diagnosis of diseases.

Abdominal Quadrants

RUQ- Right Upper Quadrant.

LUQ- Left Upper Quadrant.

RLQ- Right Lower Quadrant.

LLQ- Left Lower Quadrant.

Abdominal Regions

Right Hypochondriac

Epigastric

Left Hypochondriac

Right Lumbar

Umbilicus

Left Lumbar

Right Iliac

Hypogastric

Left Iliac

Medical Terminologies According to Abdominal Regions

Term	Word type	Origin	Meaning	Structures	Quadrant
Right Hypocho	Prefix: Hypo/Word root:	Greek	Below the Cartil	Liver, Gallbladder,	RUQ

ndriac	Chrondr/Suffix: -iac		age of the Ribs (Right side).	Right Kidney, Small Intestines.	
Epigastric	Prefix: Epi/Word root: Gastr/Suffix: -ic	Greek	Upon the Stomach or on top of the Stomach.	Stomach, Liver, Pancreas, Duodenum, Spleen, Adrenal glands.	RUQ, LUQ
Left hypochondriac	Prefix: Hypo/Word root: Chrondr/Suffix: -iac	Greek	Below the Cartilage of the Ribs (Left	Spleen, Colon, Left Kidney, Pancreas.	LUQ

			side).		
Right Lumbar	Word root: Lumb/Suffix: -ar	Latin	The right side of the Loin.	Gall bladder, Liver, right colon.	RUQ, RLQ
Umbilical	Word root: Umbilic/Suffix: -al	Latin	Of the Navel.	Umbilicus, Jejunum, Ileum, Duodenum.	RUQ, LUQ, RLQ, LLQ
Left Lumbar	Word root: Lumb/Suffix: -ar	Latin	The left side of the Loin.	Descending colon, Left Kidney.	LLQ
Right Iliac	Word root: Ili/Suffix: -ac	Latin	The right side of the	Appendix, Cecum.	RLQ

			Hips or Groin.		
Hypogastric	Prefix: Hypo/ Word root:/Gastr/ Suffix: -ic	Greek	Below the region of the Stomach.	Urinary Bladder, Sigmoid Colon, Female Reproductive Organs.	RLQ, LLQ
Left Iliac	Word root: Ili/Suffix: -ac	Latin	The left side of the Hips or Groin.	Descending Colon and Sigmoid Colon.	LLQ

Always remember:

Suffix: **-al means Pertaining to.**

Suffix: **-ic also means Pertaining to.**

Suffix: **-ar also means Pertaining to.**

Suffix: **-ac/iac also means Pertaining to.**

Quick Exercise 6

1. Human Anatomy, in simple terms, means cutting the body. True or False?
2. What do the Coronal and Sagittal body planes describe?
3. The body without the appendages is left with ______________________ and head.
4. Separate these terms into their word types: Anteroinferior, Abdominopelvic, and Thoracolumbar.

Diagnostics Investigations

Diagnosis of diseases won't be accurate without first confirming with Diagnostic tests.

Let's examine some Diagnostic investigations in Alphabetical order.

Amniocentesis- Amni/o/cente/sis: Aspiration of the Amniotic fluid for further investigation of the fetus.

Angiography- Angi/o/graphy or Arteriogram/Arteri/o/gram: A procedure involving the introduction of a radiopaque substance in other to view blood or lymph vessels. Also known as an X-ray of the blood vessels.

Anorectal Manometry- An/o/rectal/Man/o/metry: Insertion of a flexible Catheter or balloon to measure the contraction and relaxation of the Rectum and Anal Sphincter.

Arterial Blood Gas- Arter/ial/Blood/Gas: A measure of the acidity (pH), the levels of oxygen and carbon dioxide in the blood from an artery.

Arthrocentesis (Joint Aspiration)- Arthr/o/cente/sis: The Aspiration of Synovial fluids from a joint.

Arthrography- Arthr/o/graphy: Imaging of the Joints.

Audiometry- Audio/metry: Measuring hearing acuity via acoustic stimuli of frequencies.

Bacterial Analysis- Bacter/ial/Ana/lys/is: Determining the type of bacteria present in a purulent exudate.

Barium Swallow- Bar/ium/Swallow: Use of Barium and X-ray to visualize the Gastrointestinal tract.

Biopsy- Bio/o/psy: Taking a sample of body tissue for further investigation.

Bronchoscopy- Bronch/o/scopy: Insertion of a thin-lighted tube to visualize the Lungs.

Capsule Endoscopy- Capsule/End/o/scopy: Transmission of Images of the Gastrointestinal tract by ingesting a Capsule (Camera). The Camera visualizes the GI Tract.

Cardiac Catheterisation- Card/iac/Cathether/is/ation: Insertion of thin Catheter via the blood vessels to the heart to diagnose or treat Cardiac conditions.

CAT Scan: X-ray of the Kidneys in transverse form for diagnosis and treatment. (CAT- Computerised Axial Tomography)

Cervical Biopsy- Cervic/al/Bio/o/psy: Taking a sample of the Cervical tissue to diagnose Cervical conditions.

Colonoscopy- Colon/o/scopy: Insertion of a long, flexible tube via the rectum to visualize the lining of the colon for the detection of abnormalities.

Colposcopy- Colp/o/scopy: A thorough examination of the Vulva, Vagina, and Cervix using a lens.

Computed Tomography- Comput/ed/Tom/o/graphy: Crossectional images of organs using low intensity rays.

Cystopyelogram- Cyst/o/pyel/o/gram: Using ionizing radiation to view the bladder and the renal pelvis of the kidney.

Cystoscopy- Cyst/o/scopy: Insertion of flexible or rigid thin viewing tube into the bladder through the urethra.

Cytology- Cyt/o/logy: Collection of cells for study under the microscope.

Doppler flow study- Doppl/er/flow/study: Estimates blood velocity flow within the blood vessels using ultrasound waves.

Dual-energy X-ray Absorption- Du/al/Ener/gy/X-ray/Absorp/tion: Measures bone loss of hips, lumbar, and spine by using ionizing radiation in small doses to produce images.

Echocardiography- Echo/Cardi/o/graphy: The use of ultrasound waves to measure Cardiac/Heart activities for diagnosis and treatment.

Elastography- Elast/o/graghy: The use of Ultrasound and MRI to detect the elastic properties of the Liver and other soft tissues.

Electrocardiography- Electr/o/cardi/o/graphy: The use of electrodes to measure Cardiac/Heart activities for diagnosis and treatment.

Electroencephalography- Electr/o/encephal/o/graphy: The use of electrodes to measure the electrical activities of the Brain.

Electromyography- Electr/o/my/o/graphy: The use of electrodes to measure the electrical activities of the muscles in response to nerve stimulation for diagnosis and treatment.

Electronystagmography: Electr/o/nystagm/o/graphy: The use of electrodes to measure electrical activities to evaluate people with vertigo and other similar disorders.

Endometrial Biopsy: End/o/metr/ial: Taking a sample tissue of the inner lining of the uterus for further evaluation.

Endoscopic Retrograde Cholangiopancreatography-End/o/scop/ic/Retr/o/grade/Cholangi/o/pancreat/o/graphy: The injection of dye through a thin, flexible tube(endoscope) to visualize the Gastrointestinal tract (Oesophagus, Stomach, Intestines, Liver, Pancreas, and Gall bladder) with the use of an X-ray in for diagnoses and treatment.

Esophageal Manometry- Esophag/eal Man/o/metry: Insertion of a thin, flexible catheter into the Stomach through the Esophagus to ascertain the Contraction and Coordination of the Esophageal muscles.

Esophagogastroduodenoscopy-Esophag/o/gastr/o/duoden/o/scopy: Visualisation of the

Esophagus, Stomach and Duodenum through an endoscope.

Fine Needle Aspiration- Fine/Needle/Aspir/ation: Taking a sample tissue or sample fluid from a solid mass or cyst.

Fluorescence microlymphoangiography- Fluor/escence/micro/lymph/o/angi/o/graphy: The visualization of Skin lymphatics through a noninvasive method.

Fluoroscopy- Fluor/o/scopy: An imaging that continuously shows images as X-ray beams is passed through the body.

Fungal Testing- Fung/al/Testing: Observation and examination of skin scrapings from lesions to detect fungal growth.

Gonioscopy- Goni/o/scopy: Examination of the Eye's Anterior chamber for diagnosis and treatment.

Hysterosalpingography: Hyster/o/salping/o/graphy: Visualization of the Uterus and Fallopian tubes with X-rays.

Hysteroscopy- Hyster/o/scopy: Examination of the Uterus with the use of a thin telescope.

Isokinetic dynamometry- Iso/kinet/ic/Dynam/o/metry: Measurement of Muscular power with the use of a dynamometer.

Laparoscopy- Lapar/o/scopy: A surgical procedure using a keyhole incision to assess the Abdominopelvic region.

Loop Electrical Excision Procedure- Loop/Electr/ical/Excis/ion: Using Electric current via a loop wire to remove tissues in the female reproductive tract.

Lung plethysmography- Lung/plethysm/o/graphy: Measurement of lung capacity in respect to how much air it can hold.

Lymphangiography- Lymph/angi/o/graphy: Using X-ray to visualize structures of the lymphatic system by injecting a radiocontrast agent.

Lymphoscintigraphy- Lymph/o/scinti/graphy: Using gamma rays to evaluate the Lymphatic system by injecting radiotracers into the skin.

Magnetic Resonance Imaging- Magnet/ic/Reso/n/ance: Using Strong Magnetic fields and Radio waves to produce images of the body and organs.

Mammography- Mammo/graphy: Using X-rays (low energy) to examine the breast for diagnosis and treatment.

Myeolography- Myeol/o/graphy: Using contrast dye and X-ray to examine the Spinal canal for diagnosis and treatment.

Octreoscan Venous Sampling- Octre/o/scan/Venous/Sampling: A 2-day Octeotride Scan after Injection of radiocontrast through the Veins of the arm (1st day alone) to detect neuroendocrine tumors.

Ophthalmoscopy- Ophthalm/o/scopy: The examination of the interior of the eye.

Otoscopy- Oto/scopy: Use of Otoscope to examine the eye.

Pelvic ultrasound- Pelv/ic/ Ultra/sound: Using sound waves to visualize the structures in the Human pelvis for diagnosis and treatment.

Polysomnography- Poly/somn/o/graphy: Using electrodes to study and record sleep patterns and body functions during sleep for diagnosis and treatment.

Positron Emission Tomography- Posit/ron/Emiss/ion/Tom/o/graphy: Measure of the metabolic activities of body cells using nuclear energy.

Proetz test- Proetz/Test: A test to determine the acuity of smell.

Pulmonary Ventilation Perfusion Scan- Pulm/o/nary/Vent/il/ation/Per/fus/ion/Scan: Injection and inhaling of radioactive materials while Scanning the Lungs. It is a Nuclear Scan test.

Pulmonary function tests: Pulm/o/nary: These are a non-invasive group of tests that measures the functionality of the lungs.

Saline Sonography- Saline/Son/o/graphy: Using Saline solution to outline the Uterine Cavity during Ultrasound.

Sestamibi Scan: Detection of parathyroid glands via imaging for diagnosis and treatment.

Sigmoidoscopy- Sigmoid/o/scopy: Insertion of flexible or rigid thin viewing tube into the intestines through the sigmoid colon.

Thermography- Therm/o/graphy: A non-invasive procedure that detects blood flow and heat on the surface of the body through an infrared camera.

Tonometry- Ton/o/metry: Measurement of the eye pressure.

Transvaginal Ultrasonography- Trans/Vagin/al/Ultra/Son/o/graphy: Examination of the Pelvic Organs with sound waves and thin probe through the vagina.

Urinalysis- Urina/lysis: an examination of a urine sample for diagnosis and treatment.

Breaking down the complex words is the first step in memorizing and understanding these terminologies.

Surgical/Medical Interventions

Any deviation from optimum health will lead to either Medical or Surgical interventions. At times, it can lead to both. This is to ensure that the body returns to its normal or near-normal state.

Medical Terminologies According To Medical/Surgical Intervention

Abdominoperineal resection: Surgical removal of sigmoid colon, rectum, and anus through the Abdomen and pelvis.

Abdominoplasty: Surgical repair of the abdominal wall for cosmetic purpose as in tummy tuck. Plasty means Surgical repair.

Anastomosis: Surgical connection/sewing together of loops of intestines or blood vessels that are normally distant from each other.

Anoplasty: Surgical procedure involving repair of the anus.

Appendectomy: Surgical Excision of the appendix.

Balanoplasty: Surgical repair of the glans penis.

Blepharoplasty: Surgical repair of the upper and lower eyelids for reduction.

Brachioplasty: Surgical repair of the upper arms and part of the armpit (axillae) for reduction as in Arm lift.

Brachytherapy: A treatment that involves introducing radioactive seeds on malignant prostate cells.

Bullectomy: Surgical removal of damaged air sacs from the lungs. Commonly found in patients with Chronic Obstructive Pulmonary Disease.

Cardiac Ablation: Use of radio-frequency to destroy heart tissues causing abnormal rhythm.

Cataract surgery: Surgical procedure to remove cloudy lens and replace with an artificial one.

Cesarean section: A surgical procedure involving removal of the fetus from the uterus through the abdominal wall.

Cholecystectomy: Surgical Excision of the gallbladder.

Circumcision: Surgical incision or cutting around of the foreskin of the glans penis.

Colectomy: Surgical removal of the colon.

Colostomy: Surgical opening through the abdominal wall into the colon.

Colpopexy: Surgical procedure involving the fixation of the vagina.

Cool Sculpting (Cryolipolysis): Non-invasive procedure to freeze and dissolve adipose tissue under the skin for cosmetic purposes.

Core decompression: Removing the Central part of a diseased bone and filling the area with bone graft.

Craniectomy: Surgical removal of a portion of the skull to allow brain swelling to resolve and fix it back with a second surgery.

Craniotomy: Surgical procedure involving removal of part of the skull to expose the brain for further surgery.

Cryoextraction of a cataract: Removal of a cloudy lens through a cold probe.

Cryotherapy: A treatment that involves destroying body tissues with liquid nitrogen.

Cystectomy: Excision of the bladder.

Cystoplasty: Surgical procedure involving repair of the bladder.

Cystostomy: Surgical procedure that involves creating an opening into the bladder.

Cystotomy: Surgical cutting into the bladder.

Debridement: Surgical removal of damaged, dead and infected tissue from the skin or wound surface to promote healing.

Decortication of the lung: Procedure to remove fibrous tissues abnormally formed on the Lung surface.

Dermabrasion: The process of scraping away the epidermis of the skin to reveal new ones or get rid of damaged ones.

Dermatoplasty: Surgical repair or reconstruction of the skin to repair damaged skin.

Diathermy: Use of High-frequency energy current that produces heat for Surgical procedures and Physical therapies. Dia means through, and Therm means heating.

Electrolysis: Using electricity to destroy and dissolve body tissues, as in the removal of hair.

Endotracheal intubation: Procedure used to establish airway by inserting a tube into the lungs via the trachea.

Enucleation: Procedure to Surgically remove the eyes.

Episiotomy: Surgical cutting into the perineum to allow more space for the fetus.

Facelift/Rhytidectomy: Surgical procedure involving the removal of Facial skin, fat, and muscle to lessen signs of aging.

Fasciectomy: Surgical incision into the muscle to remove the fascia (fibrous band).

Fasciodesis: Surgical binding of a fibrous band of a muscle to a tendon. Desis means Binding together.

Fasciotomy: Surgical incision into the fascia.

Fenestration: Surgical procedure that involves creating an opening into a Visceral.

Gastrectomy: Surgical removal of the stomach.

Gastrojejunostomy: Surgical opening between the jejunum of the small intestine and the stomach.

Gastrostomy: Surgical opening into the stomach through the abdominal wall for feeding.

Hemodialysis: A procedure involving filtration of wastes and water from the blood via a machine.

Herniorrhaphy: Surgical repair of hernia by suturing.

Hymenectomy: Surgical removal of the hymen.

Hypophysectomy: Excision of the pituitary gland.

Hysterectomy: Excision of the Uterus — through the abdomen or vagina.

Hysteropexy: Surgical procedure involving fixation of the uterus to stabilize it.

Ileostomy: Surgical opening into the ileum.

Incision and drainage: Surgical procedure that involves cutting into an abscess and draining out the content.

Jejunostomy: Surgical opening into the jejunum.

Keratoplasty: Surgical repair of the cornea by replacing the affected cornea with a normal one.

Labyrinthectomy: Surgical procedure that involves removal of the Labyrinth.

Laminectomy: Excision of the lamina of the spinal column to release pressure on the spinal cord. Lamina means Plates of bones covering the vertebrae.

Laparoscopic adjustable gastric band: An incision into the stomach to place an adjustable strap/band around the stomach to induce weight loss.

Laser Angioplasty: Use of laser beams to open blocked coronary arteries.

Laser photocoagulation: Use of laser beam to destroy leaking or damaged vessels in the eye in cases of senile degeneration and diabetic retinopathy.

Laser therapy: Use of intense light to cut and destroy tissues, particularly damaged skin tissues (LASER means Light Amplification by Stimulated Emission of Radiation).

Laser-assisted in situ keratomileusis: Use of Laser beams to correct eye deficiencies.

Liposuction: Surgical procedure involving suction of subcutaneous fat.

Lipotripsy: Non- invasive procedure that involves crushing of body fat. Tripsy means Crushing.

Lobectomy: Surgical removal/Excision of the Lobe of the lung.

Lumpectomy: Surgical procedure involving removal of lump only from the breast.

Lung Volume Reduction Surgery: An open chest surgery involving the removal of a diseased part of an inflated lung for the functional one to grow.

Lung transplantation: Replacement of damaged lungs from a compatible donor; it can be one or both lungs.

Mastectomy: Surgical procedure involving removal of the breast(s) or breast tissues. It can be simple or total/radical.

Mastoidectomy: Surgical procedure that involves removal of mastoid air cells.

Mastoidotomy: Surgical incision into the mastoid bone.

Meniscectomy: Excision of the Meniscus of the knee. Tomy means Incision/Excision/Cutting, and Meniscus is a cartilage in the knee that helps to stabilize the joint and lubricate the knee.

Meniscopexy: Surgical procedure to fix the Meniscus. Pexy means Fixation.

Metatarsal arthroplasty: Surgical repair of the joint of the big toe, usually used in the treatment of Arthritis.

Myolysis: Surgical procedure to loosen or dissolve a muscle. Lysis means Loosened or dissolved.

Myomectomy: Excision of a leiomyoma from the uterus.

Myoplasty: Surgical procedure to repair a muscle.

Myorrhaphy: Procedure involving Suturing of the muscle.

Myringoplasty: Surgical procedure that involves repair of the tympanic membrane.

Myringotomy: Surgical incision into the tympanic membrane.

Nephrectomy: Surgical removal of the kidney(s).

Nephrolithotomy: Surgical removal of kidney stones.

Nerve ablation: Destruction of the nerves usually as a result of pain. Ablation means Destruction.

Neurectomy: Surgical procedure to remove a nerve.

Neuroplasty: Surgical procedure to repair a nerve.

Oophorectomy: Excision of an ovary.

Orchidectomy: Excision of one or both testes.

Orchidopexy: Surgical procedure involving the fixation of a testicle.

Orchioplasty: Surgical procedure involving the repair of the testis.

Osteoclasis: Surgical procedure to break the bone to correct a malformation. Osteo means bone, while Clasis means to break.

Osteoplasty: Surgical procedure to repair the bone.

Osteotomy: Surgical cutting or Incision to the bone. Tomy means Cutting or Incision.

Patellectomy: Surgical cutting into the knee to remove the Patella.

Penile implant: Surgical implantation of a prosthesis into the penis.

Percutaneous transluminal coronary angioplasty (PTCA): Insertion of a balloon catheter into a blood vessel to flatten a plaque against its wall for blood flow to resume.

Phacoemulsification of cataract: Use of ultrasonic vibration to dissolve the portions of the lens and also aspirate the broken structures of the cornea.

Phalangectomy: Surgical cutting into the Phalanges to remove a finger or toe.

Photoreactive keratectomy: Use of laser beam to restructure the cornea.

Pleurocentesis: A surgical procedure involves puncture of the pleural space to drain fluids.

Pneumonectomy: Surgical procedure involving removal or excision of the lung(s).

Polypectomy: Surgical excision of the polyps in the colon.

Prostatectomy: Excision of the prostate gland.

Pyloroplasty: Surgical procedure involving repair of the pylorus of the stomach.

Renal transplant: Surgical replacement of the diseased Kidney by a compatible, healthy donor.

Salpingectomy: Excision of the fallopian tube(s).

Salpingo-oophorectomy: Excision of the fallopian tubes and ovaries.

Scleroplasty: Surgical repair of the sclera.

Sclerotherapy: A treatment that involves shrinkage or closing off of the veins by introducing a sclerosing agent as in varicose veins.

Small Incision lenticule extraction: Procedure to correct multiple refractive errors by making a small cut into the side of the cornea and extracting the lenticule using microforceps. Lenticle means Disc-shaped cornea tissue.

Stapedectomy: Surgical removal of the staples of the ear.

Stent Insertion: A procedure that follows PTCA, involving the application of a mesh-like substance to keep the vessel always open.

Tenodesis: Surgical binding or fixation of a tendon.

Tenomyoplasty: Surgical procedure to repair the Muscle and Tendon.

Tenorrhaphy: Procedure involving Suturing of the tendon. The suffix "rrhaphy" means Suturing.

Tenotomy: Surgical incision into the tendon.

Thoracocentesis: An invasive procedure involving puncturing the chest wall or thorax via a canular to drain accumulated fluids or expel air. Centesis means to Puncture.

Thoracotomy: Surgical incision into the thorax or chest wall.

Total hip replacement arthroplasty: Replacement of the head of femur and hip joint with a metallic femoral head and plastic acetabulum. Arthro means Joint, Plasty means Surgical repair.

Total hysterectomy and bilateral salpingo-oophorectomy: Surgical removal of the uterus and cervix, both fallopian tubes with their ovaries.

Total knee joint replacement arthroplasty: Replacement of the knee joint with prostheses. Arthro means Joint, while Plasty means Surgical repair.

Tympanectomy: Excision of the tympanic membrane (Eardrum).

Tympanoplasty: Surgical repair of the tympanic membrane (Eardrum).

Unicompartmental hip/knee resurfacing: An alternative to total knee replacement, Only the affected knee is resurfaced.

Urethropexy: Surgical procedure involving fixation of the urethra.

Uvulectomy: Excision of part or all of the uvula following obstructive sleep apnea.

Uvulopalatopharyngoplasty: Surgical procedure involving repair of the Uvula, Palate, and Pharynx.

Vaginoplasty: Surgical procedure involving repair of the vagina.

Vagotomy: Surgical removal of part or all of the vagus nerve.

Varicocelectomy: Excision of a varicocele.

Vasectomy: Surgical removal of a part of the vas deferens as a contraceptive.

Vasoepididymostomy: Surgical procedure involving joining of vas deferens and epididymis as a measure to infertility.

Ventriculoperitoneal shunting: Surgical procedure to drain excess fluid from the ventricles of the brain, which is directed to other parts of the body.

Vitrectomy: Surgical procedure to replace the vitreous humor of the eye.

Vulvectomy: Excision of the external genitalia.

Pharmacology

Pharmacology is from the Greek word Pharmako — **Medicine** — and logy — **Study of.** You'll be correct to say Pharmacology is the study of medicine (drugs) but not only the study of medicine but also the study of the interaction these drugs have between themselves and the human body.

Over time, the method of administering medications has evolved. We now have more advanced and faster routes to make drugs work in the body, with no more limitations to the oral route. Below are some of the various routes of administration to ensure patients get their doses.

Oral route

Buccal or sublingual

Parenteral route (intravenous, intramuscular, intradermal, subcutaneous)

Transdermal

Topical route

Ocular route

Rectal route

Vagina route

Otic route

Nasal route

Intrathecal route

Intracardiac route

Inhalation/ pulmonary route

These routes ensure that medications are given at precise rates. Check out some of the common medications used in practice.

Balanced Salt Solution: A solution slightly different from normal saline in the composition used to wash out the eye. (Also known as BSS)

Beta-blockers: Used in the treatment of cardiovascular diseases, they block the effect of epinephrine, causing the heart to beat slower and consequently lowering blood pressure. Also used in the treatment of Glaucoma because of the effects on pressure. **Metoprolol, Propanolol, Atenolol,** and **Carvedilol.**

Mydriatic drugs: Used to dilate the pupil of the eyes. It can be used during an eye examination. **Paremyd, Prefrin, Isopto Homatropine,** and **Cyclogyl.**

Prostaglandin analogs: They are Ocular hypotensive drugs used in the treatment of Glaucoma. **Latanoprost, Bimatropost, Travopost,** and **Bimatropost ophthalmic implant.**

Silver nitrate: Topical anti-infective agent.

Angiotensin-converting enzyme (ACE) inhibitors: They lower blood pressure by enlarging and dilating blood vessels due to their inhibition property on the enzyme ACE. **Benazepril**, **Captopril, Enalapril, Fosinopril, Lisinopril,** and **Ramipril.**

Aldosterone antagonist: Antagonizes the action of aldosterone, thereby acting as a Diuretic. Used in the treatment of cardiovascular diseases. **Spironolactone, Aldactone, Finerenone, CapoSpril,** and **Eplerenone.**

Antiarrhythmics: Suppresses Abnormal rhythms and Conducting of the heart. **Amiodarone, Flecainide, Ibutilide,** and **Lidocaine.**

Anticoagulants: Suppresses blood clotting ability. **Rivaroxaban, Heparin, Warfarin, Enoxaparin,** and **Edoxaban.**

Calcium channel blockers: Blocks calcium from entering blood vessels and cells, causing blood pressure to be lowered. They can also be used in the treatment of Angina Pectoris and Cardiac Arrhythmias **Amlodipine, Nifedipine, Verapamil, Felodipine,** and **Nicardipine hydrochloride.**

Lipid-lowering agents: Used to lower blood lipid. **Bile acid resins, Nicotinic acid, Omega 3 fatty acids,** and **fatty esters.**

Bronchodilators Used to increase airflow to the lungs by decreasing respiratory resistance and improving respiration. **Salbutamol, Theophylline,** and **Ipratropium.**

Corticosteroids (Man-made steroids): reduce inflammation. **Prednisolone**, **Methylprednisolone**, **Dexamethasone, Betamethasone**, and **Hydrocortisone**.

Diuretics: Drugs that increase the excretion of water and salt from the body. They are excreted by the kidneys.

Bumetanide, Ethacrynic acid, Furosemide, and **Torsemide.**

Antitussives: Drugs that suppress coughing reflex in the brain. **Dextromethorphan Benzonatate, Codeine.**

Expectorants: They loosen mucus in the Upper and Lower Respiratory tract. **Guaifenesin, Potassium iodide.**

Antibiotics: They destroy or slow the growth of bacteria, causing diseases in the body. **Amoxicillin, Azithromycin, Amoxicillin/Clavulanate, Clindamycin, Cephalexin,** and **Ciprofloxacin.**

Anticholinergics: They block the action of a neurotransmitter- acetylcholine, thereby inhibiting the parasympathetic nervous system. **Atropine, Belladonna alkaloids, Benztropine mesylate, Clidinium, Cyclopentolate, Darifenacin,** and **Dicyclomine.**

Histamine 2 blockers: Reduces the amount of Gastric acid secretion. **Cimetidine, Famotidine**, **Nizatidine,** and **Ranitidine.**

Emetics: Drugs that induce vomiting. **Apomorphine, Cupric sulfate,** and **Ipecac.**

Antiemetics: Drugs that stop the action of vomiting. **Diphenhydramine, Metoclopramide, Promethazine,** and **Ondansetron.**

Proton pump inhibitors: Reduces the amount of Gastric acid production. **Rabeprazole, Omeprazole, Esomeprazole,** and **Lansoprazole.**

Activated Charcoal: Used in the treatment of poisons as it is known for its absorbing properties

Antiresorptive: Used in the treatment of Osteoporosis to slow down bone loss. **Alendronate, Risedronate.**

Anti-Gouts: Increases the excretion of uric acid via the kidneys and reduces the production of uric acid by the body. **Allopurinol, Probenecid.**

Disease-modifying antirheumatic drugs: Used in the management of Rheumatoid arthritis. **Methotrexate, Hydroxychloroquine,** and **Sulfasalazine.**

Anti-neuropathic pain medications: Used to reduce nerve pain caused by injuries or dysfunctions. **Pregabalin, Amitriptyline.**

Nonsteroidal anti-inflammatory drugs: Used to treat pain associated with inflammation, fever, and blood clot. **Diclofenac, Ibuprofen,** and **Aspirin, Celecoxib.**

Capsaicin: Interferes between the nerve pain signal and the brain. Contains Chilli and is used in the treatment of musculoskeletal disorders.

Opioid analgesics: Acts on opioid receptors to relieve pain and also has an anesthetic effect. **Tramadol, Morphine, Codeine,** and **Fentanyl.**

Non-narcotic analgesics: Used to relieve pain, is short-acting and does not possess anesthetic properties. **NSAIDs, Acetaminophen.**

Thyroid and Antithyroid Agents: Used in the treatment of Thyroid associated diseases. **Carbimazole, Methimazole, and Propylthiouracil, Levothyroxine (T4),** and **Liothyronine (T3).**

Hypoglycemic Agents: Used to decrease the level of glucose in the blood. **Glimepiride, Repaglinide, Metformin, Pioglitazone,** and **Sitagliptin.**

Insulin, Long-Acting: Parenteral medications are used to decrease the glucose level in the blood. **Insulin lispro /**

insulin lispro protamine, insulin inhalation, rapid-acting, and **insulin aspart / insulin aspart protamine.**

Reproductive hormonal drugs: **Dihydrotestosterone, Estradiol,** and **Progesterone.**

Anticonvulsants: Used in the treatment of epilepsy and seizure. Also, act as mood stabilizers. **Gabapentin, Levetiracetam, Carbamazepine,** and **Phenobarbital.**

Hypnotics/Sedatives: Psychoactive drugs are used to create calm effects and induce sleep

and sedation. **Zolpidem, Triazolam, Estazolam,** and **Cloroqualone.**

Central nervous system stimulants: Used to increase CNS activities by increasing the number of neurochemicals in the brain. **Dextroamphetamine, Methylphenidate, Doxapram,** and **Caffeine.**

Drugs used in the treatment of Sexually transmitted infections: **Azithromycin Ceftriaxone, Ciprofloxacin Penicillin Acyclovir, Valacyclovir,** and **Famciclovir.** In the treatment of Human Immunodeficiency Virus - **Zidovudine, Abacavir, Lamivudine, Etravirine,** and **Atazanavir.**

Drugs used in the treatment of Cancer: **5-FU (Fluorouracil Injection), Acalabrutinib, Bexarotene, Chlorambucil,** and **Trabectedin.**

Quick Exercise 7

1. The difference between Laparoscopy and Laparotomy is ________________.

2. LASER means ______________.

3. Pharmacology is of Latin origin. True or False?

4. Anti-Gout medications prevent the production of uric acids by the body. List them.

Acronyms And Abbreviations

ABG - Arterial blood gas

ACE- Angiotensin-converting enzyme

ADH - Antidiuretic hormones

ADL- Activities of daily living

AED - Automated external defibrillator

AIDS - Acquired Immunodeficiency Syndrome

AKA- Above-knee amputation

AKI - Acute kidney injury

AMA - Against medical advice

AP- Angina Pectoris

ARDS - Acute respiratory distress syndrome

ARM- Artificial rupture of membranes

ART - Assisted Reproductive Technology

AV- Atrioventricular valve

BCG - Bacillus Calmette Guerin

BP - Blood pressure

BPH - Benin prostate hyperplasia

BS - Blood sugar

BSO - Bilateral salpingo-oophorectomy

BUN - Blood urea nitrogen

C-Section - Cesarean Section

C/o - Complains of

CAT - Computed axial tomography

CBC - Complete blood count

CO - Carbon monoxide

COPD - Chronic obstructive pulmonary disease

CPAP - Continuous positive airway pressure

CPR - Cardiopulmonary resuscitation

CVS - Chorionic villus sampling

CXR - Chest x-ray

Chemo - Chemotherapy

D/S - Dextrose in saline

D/W - Dextrose in water

DC - Discontinue

DEXA - Dual-energy X-ray absorptiometry

DIC - Diffuse intravascular coagulation

DM - Diabetes Mellitus

DNA - Deoxyribonucleic acid

DVT - Deep vein thrombosis

Diff - Differential blood count

Dx - Diagnosis

EBL - Estimated blood loss

ECG - Electrocardiogram

ECHO - Echocardiogram

ECT - Electroconvulsive therapy

EDD - Expected date of delivery

EEG - Electroencephalography

EGD - Esophagogastroduodenoscopy

ENT - Ear, nose, and throat

ER - Emergency room

ERCP - Endoscopic Retrograde cholangiopancreatography

FAS - Fetal alcoholic Syndrome

FOBT- Fetal occult blood test

FSH - Follicle-stimulating hormone

GERD - Gastroesophageal reflux disease

GH - Growth hormone

GI - Gastrointestinal

GSW - Gunshot wound

H&H - Hemoglobin and Hematocrit

HBV - Hepatitis B virus

HCL - Hydrochloric acid

HD - Hemodialysis

HHD - Hypertensive heart disease

HIV - Human immunodeficiency virus

HRT - Hormone replacement therapy

HTN - Hypertension

Hx - History

I&D - Incision and drainage

I&O - Intake and Output

IBS - Irritable bowel syndrome

ICU - Intensive care unit

IM - Intramuscular

IUD - Intrauterine device

IV - Intravenous

KIV - Keep in view

KVO - Keep vein open

LASIK - Laser-assisted in situ keratomileusis

LEEP - Loop electrosurgical excision procedure

LVRS - Lung volume reduction surgery

MCS - Microscopic culture and sensitivity

MD - Medical Doctor

MI- Myocardial infarction

MRA - Magnetic resonance angiography

MRI - Magnetic resonance imaging

MS - Multiple sclerosis

MVP - Mitral valve prolapse

NG - Nasogastric

NICU - Neonatal intensive care unit

NIDDM - Non-insulin-dependent diabetes mellitus

NPO - Nil per oral

OB/GYN - Obstetrics and gynecology

OP - Outpatient

OR - Operating room

ORIF - Open reduction internal fixation

OSA - Obstructive sleep apnea

PCOS - polycystic ovarian syndrome

PCV - Packed cell volume

PE - Pulmonary embolism

PEG - Percutaneous endoscopic gastrostomy

PET - Positron emission tomography

PFT - Pulmonary function test

PICU - Pediatric intensive care unit

PID - Pelvic inflammatory disease

PIH - Pregnancy-induced hypertension

PTSD - Post-traumatic stress disorder

PVD - Peripheral Vascular disease

Pap smear - Papanicolaou smear

Px - Prognosis

RDS - Respiratory distress syndrome

ROM - Range of motion

Rx - Prescription

SAB - Spontaneous Abortion

SARS - Severe acute respiratory syndrome

SBE - Self-breast examination

SCA - Sudden cardiac arrest

SIDS - Sudden infant death syndrome

SLE - systemic lupus erythematous

SMILE - Small incision lenticule extraction

Stat - Immediately

STD - Sexually transmitted diseases

STI - Sexually transmitted infection

TAB - Therapeutic abortion

TAH - Total abdominal hysterectomy

TAH/BSO - Total abdominal hysterectomy/bilateral salpingo-oophorectomy

THA - Total hip arthroplasty

THR - Total hip replacement

TPN - Total parenteral nutrition

Tx - Treatment

UPPP - Uvulopalatopharyngoplasty

UTI - Urinary tract infection

VBAC - Vaginal birth after Cesarean section

Eponyms; Named after who?

Take note of these names

Penrose drain - Charles Bingham PENROSE (1890)

Pouch of Douglas - DOUGLAS, James (1730)

Menière's disease - MENIÈRE, Prosper (1861)

Goodpasture syndrome - GOODPASTURE, Ernest William (1919)

Foley Catheter - FOLEY, Frederic Eugene Basil (1929)

Ryle nasogastric tube - RYLE, John Alfred (1921)

Yankauer mask (1904); Yankauer suction catheter (1907); Yankauer laryngeal medicator (1907); Yankauer operation (1910); Yankauer Speculum (1911); Yankauer surgical instruments (1917) - YANKAUER, Sidney (1904, 1907, 1907, 1910, 1911, 1917)

Muller sign - MÜLLER, Friedrich von (1889)

Guillain-Barré syndrome - BARRÉ, Jean-Alexandre and GUILLAIN, Georges Charles (1916)

Fournier gangrene - FOURNIER, Jean-Alfred (1883)

Cotard Syndrome - COTARD, Jules (1882)

Burns ligament - BURNS, Allan (1802)

Fleischner Sign - FLEISCHNER, Felix G (1959)

Willis-Ekbom syndrome (Restless Leg Syndrome), Ekbom syndrome II (Delusional parasitosis) - EKBOM, Karl-Axel (1944, 1938)

APGAR score - APGAR, Virginia (1953)

Battle sign - BATTLE, William Henry Marfleet (1890)

Stevens-Johnson syndrome - STEVENS, Albert Mason and JOHNSON, Frank Chambliss (1922)

Bell's palsy - BELL, Sir Charles (1827)

Graves disease - GRAVES, Robert James (1835)

Andersen disease - ANDERSEN, Dorothy Hansine (1956)

Purkinje fibers - PURKINJE, Jan Evangelista (1845)

Whipple procedure - WHIPPLE, Allen Oldfather (1934)

Hirschsprung disease - HIRSCHSPRUNG, Harald (1886)

Ringers solution - RINGER, Sidney (1882)

Hartmann solution - HARTMANN, Alexis Frank (1932)

Ortolani test - ORTOLANI, Marino (1936)

Cheyne-Stokes Respiration - STOKES, William and CHEYNE, John (1818, 1854)

Alzheimer's disease - ALZHEIMER Alois (1906)

Cushing's syndrome - CUSHING Williams Harvey (1932)

Down's syndrome - DOWN John Haydon (1866)

Parkinson's disease - PARKINSON James (1817)

Pluralizing Suffixes

When it comes to turning a single medical term into a plural, English rules are overruled. These are basic ten rules to follow:

1st Rule: Replacing “um” with “a.”

Flagell**um** - Flagell**a**

Bacteri**um** - Bacteri**a**

2nd Rule: Replacing “us” with “i.”

Bronch**us** - Bronch**i**

Pylor**us** - Pylor**i**

3rd Rule: Adding “e” to “a.”

Axill**a** - Axilla**e**

Choler**a** - Cholera**e**

4th Rule: Replacing “is” with “es.”

Stenos**is** - Stenos**es**

Prognos**is** - Prognos**es**

5th Rule: Replacing “itis” with “itides.”

Mening**itis** - Mening**itides**

Arthr**itis** - Arthr**itides**

6th Rule: Replacing “y” with “ies.”

Arter**y** - Arter**ies**

Therap**y** - Therap**ies**

7th Rule: Replacing “nx” with “nges.”

Phala**nx** - Phala**nges**

Lary**nx** - Lary**nges**

8th Rule: Replacing “x” with “ces.”

Corte**x** - Corti**ces**

Caly**x** - Cali**ces**

9th Rule: Replacing “ma” or “oma” with “mata.”

Sarco**ma** - Sarco**mata**

Leiomyo**ma** - Leiomyo**mata**

10th Rule: Replacing “on” with “a.”

Spermatozo**on** - Spermatozo**a**

Criteri**on** - Criteri**a**

Other rules include:

Pluralizing Latin words that have both nouns and adjectives.

Abruptio Placentae

Chrondromalacia Patellae

Adding "s" at the end of the term.

Chorions

Forceps

Homonyms And Synonyms

Some medical terms sound alike, although they possess different meanings. In the same vein, there are words with entirely different spelling and pronunciation with similar meanings.

Let's examine a few Homonyms.

Callous and Callus

Callous - Cold towards someone.

Callus - A thick and hardened area of the skin.

Carotid and Parotid

Carotid - An artery in the neck.

Parotid - Salivary gland in the mouth.

Fecal and Cecal

Fecal: As in feces, e.g., Fecal compaction.

Cecal: As in cecum of the intestine.

Poly and Holy

Poly: Many.

Holy: Set apart.

Ilium and Ileum

Ilium: A pelvic bone.

Ileum: part of the intestine.

Gastrotomy and Gastrostomy

Gastrotomy: Surgical incision into the stomach.

Gastrostomy: An artificial opening into the stomach.

Synonyms

Dead/Expired: To cease to have life.

Excision/Removal: To take away from.

Anterior/In front: Before.

Medication/Drugs: Medicine.

Prophylaxis/Preventive: Not allowing to occur.

Sedative/Hypnotic: Exerting a calming effect.

Quick Exercise 8

1. Give the full meaning of these abbreviations: PTSD, CAT, TAH, and CBC.
2. APGAR score was discovered by who in what year?
3. Rewrite these terminologies in their Plural forms using the rules above; Acetabulum, Appendix, and Coccus.

CHAPTER 5
ORGANISATION OF LIFE

You have learned much knowledge from the previous chapters, including the body's anatomy and many more. This chapter will examine the organization of life, the origin of humans, and how they interact with their environment. This is particularly important for listening, assessing, diagnosing, and treating patients and clients in everyday practice. This chapter will also focus on Medical terminologies according to the body systems, their physiology, and some diseases that pertain to them.

The role of physiology in the study of medicine can never be overemphasized. It deals with the normal function of your body, so imagine how essential this aspect is. Its focus is on how the body is organized from the simplest to the most complex; these include the organelles, cells, tissues, organs, and system; how they work in carrying out their chemical and physical functions. Also, the community you live in, the population, the biosphere, and the entire ecosystem play an important role in the organization of your life.

Below is a brief explanation of how human life is organized from the smallest cell to the complex system and the ecosystem.

The Organelles

They are substances that function to keep the cell alive by performing various operations in the cell.

The Cell

They are the smallest structural unit of a living organism. They have organelles that perform various tasks in them.

The Tissues

A group of cells with similar structures come together to form the tissue. There are four types of cells in the body: connective, epithelial, muscle, and nervous, and each perform a specific function.

The Organs

A Group of tissues with similar structures and functions come together to form an organ. Examples of organs include the kidney, liver, pancreas, etc.

The System

A Group of organs comes together to form a system, e.g., the digestive system, integumentary system, reproductive system, etc.

The Organism

An organism is a living creature that comes together and makes an individual entity like you, me, and everybody around us.

Community

This group of people come together and live in the same place, sharing some common characteristics.

Population

This is a group of people living together with common characteristics or features.

Ecosystem

This is an area where plants and animals occupy and form a bubble of life.

As stated earlier, many systems come together and provide normal functions in the body.

These systems include:

- Integumentary system
- Respiratory system
- Circulatory system
- Digestive system
- Reproductive system
- Nervous system
- Lymphatic system
- Endocrine system
- Urinary system
- Musculoskeletal system
- Special senses

Each system will be examined, but before that, here are some important medical technologies according to the body systems.

Medical Technologies According to The Integumentary System

The integumentary system (the word integumentary means covering) is the largest in the body, and it consists of the skin and its appendages, certain glands, hairs, and nails. It accounts for 15% of the body weight. And covers an area with a diameter of 10¾ to 21½ ft^2. The integumentary system functions in homeostasis; the maintenance of the normal internal environment of the body, it protects the body against disease and infections, serves as a way of eliminating waste products from the body through sweating, and overall regulates the temperature in the body.

The integumentary system consists of many layers, tissues, and glands.

The EPIDERMIS is the first layer of the skin that is cellular and composed of epithelium. It doesn't have blood vessels, connective tissue, cartilage, fat or lymphatic vessels.

The Dermis

The dermis is the second layer of the skin below the epidermis. It is also called CORIUM. The dermis contains blood vessels, connective tissues, lymphatic vessels, and other substances absent in the epidermis, which makes it different from the epidermis.

Subcutaneous Layer

This layer of the skin consists of the connective tissues that aid the formation of fats. It's an important layer of the skin that concerns the protection and acts as a heat insulator.

Terminologies	Combining Form	Vowel	Meaning	Example
Adip	Adip(o)	O	Fat	In the case of adipose tissues, that lies three layers deep under the skin. Its main function is storing lipid and triglycerides.

Aut	Aut(o)	O	Self	
Bi	Bi(o)	O	Life	
Blephar	Blephar(o)	O	Eyelid	
Albino	Albin(o)	O	White	Just in the case of people with a lack of skin pigmentation.
Carcin	Carcin(o)	O	Carcino ma	
Cutane	Cutane(o)	O	Skin	In case of something related to the skin or something that affects

				the skin.
Cyan	Cyan(o)	O	Blue	In the case of cyanosis, a condition characterized by the bluish coloration of the skin.
Dermat	Dermat(o)	O	Skin	Dermatology, branch of medicine that deals with skin and its components.
Derm	Derm(o)	O	Skin	It means skin, just like in the case of a dermatologist, skin

				specialist.
Diaphor	Diaphor(o)	O		
Erythem	Erythem(o)	O	Red	Just like in the case of erythema, a condition characterized by redness of the skin.
Hidr	Hidr(o)	O	Sweat	
Histi	Histi(o)	O	Tissue	
Icter	Icter(o)	O	Yellow	Like in the case of icterus, also known as jaundice, a condition

				characterized by the yellowish coloration of the skin and tissues.
Integument	Integumen t(o)	O	Skin	The integumentary system.
Kerat	Kerat(o)	O	Hard	
Leuk	Leuk(o)	O	White	In the case of Leukocytes, also known as white blood cells that defend against infection and diseases.

Lip	Lip(o)	O	Fat	Lipid; an insoluble substance and the most constituents of plant and animal cells.
Melan	Melan(o)	O	Black	Melanin; forms from melanocytes; it's a skin pigment.
Onych	Onych(o)	O	Nail	In the case of Onychodystrophy, a condition characterized by abnormal growth of the nails.

Papil	Papil(o)	O	Nippleli ke	
Pil	Pil(o)	O	Hair	
Py	Py(o)	O	Pus	
Rhytid	Rhytid(o)	O	Wrinkle	
Sclera	Sclera(o)	O	Hardeni ng	In the case of scleroderma, a condition characterized by hardening of the skin.
Seb	Seb(o)	O	Fat	
Squam	Squam(o)	O	Scale	

Streat	Streat(o)	O	Fat	
Trich	Trich(o)	O	Hair	
Xanth	Xanth(o)	O	Yellow	Xanthoma; a condition characterized by the building of fats under the surface of the skin.
Xer	Xer(o)	O	Dry	The condition of xerosis, also known as dry skin; a continuous characterized by the roughness of dryness of the

				skin.

Some common integumentary diseases and their pharmacology treatments.

The conditions that affect the skin are sometimes obvious and troublesome; they include;

Ance: A condition characterized by the inflammation of the skin, and the most common is acne vulgaris, and it can be treated with some over the counter medicine

Bulla: a condition characterized by blisters in the skin. This can be treated with some antibiotics like dicloxacillin, cephalexin, clindamycin, etc.

Carbuncle: the presence of blackheads or keratin in a skin pore. This condition can be treated with a simple incision or drainage.

Comedo: blackheads that are caused by sebum or keratin buildup in a skin pore. Treatment for this disease can be done using some cleansers like salicylic acid or gentle exfoliate with AHAs (Alpha hydroxy acid) and BHAs (Beta hydroxy acid).

Papule: a condition characterized by a solid elevation of the skin. The condition can be treated with retinoids or retinoids like drugs or with antibiotics.

Ulcer: an erosion in the skin. Treatment for this includes; corticotherapy, dapsone, clofazimine, and cyclosporine.

Keloid: an abnormal thickening of a scar. Pharmacological treatments for this disease include using growth factors, immunomodulators, anti-allergy, and anti-inflammatory drugs.

Urticaria: a condition characterized by hives with swelling and itching in the skin. The main treatment for this disease is second-generation oral antihistamines, e.g., loratadine, desloratadine, or fexofenadine.

Vitiligo: a condition characterized by white patches in the skin due to loss of pigment. The treatment for this abnormality is topical corticosteroids.

Medical Terminologies According to The Respiratory System

The RESPIRATORY system is another important system in the body's normal function — breathing, which indicates being alive. The respiratory system's primary function is to provide oxygen for the body's normal function and eliminate carbon dioxide. Internal respiration is the exchange of gases from the lungs to the other organs in the body. External respiration is the exchange of gases between the external environment and the lungs.

Aside from the lungs, many organs also participate in the action of respiration.

They include; the nose, the pharynx, the larynx, the trachea, and the bronchi. Each of them plays a vital role in keeping organisms alive and healthy.

The Nose or Nasal Cavity

This is the first organ, and the first process of respiration occurs here. When the oxygen is inhaled, it is through the nasal cavity that the oxygen enters the body. The nose is also a means of protection in the body; it contains mucous membranes and hairs called cilia that trap foreign bodies from entering your body. The nasal cavity also moistens and warms the air that enters.

The Pharynx and Larynx

Air passes through the nose to the Pharynx, and the pharynx consists of three layers, the nasopharynx, oropharynx, and hypopharynx. The last layer of the pharynx is what gives rise to the larynx and the esophagus. The larynx leads to the trachea, and from there, the air is passed to the lungs.

Trachea

When air passes through the larynx, it enters the trachea, and from there, it reaches the bronchi.

Bronchi

The trachea bifurcates and gives rise to the bronchi, and each of these bronchi separately enters each.

Below are some made easy medical terminologies according to the respiratory system.

Terminologies	Combining Form	Vowel	Meaning	Example
Aer	Aer(o)	O	Air	Just in the case of Aerodrome

				from airdrome. Which is a place from which aircraft flight operations take place.
Atel	Atel(o)	O	Imperfect	For example, atelophobia: a situation where people are scared of imperfectio n.
Bronch	Bronch(o)	O	Bronchus	The bronchus, which is a

				singular word, is a tube that carries oxygen to the lungs.
Bronchiol	Bronchiol (o)	O	Bronchiol es	The bronchioles are inside the lungs; they deliver air to alveoli, where gaseous exchange occurs.
Laryng	Laryng(o)	O	Larynx	Also called the voice box, it helps in breathing

				and prevents food particles from entering the trachea.
Lob	Lob(o)	O	Lobes	Just in the case of the lobes that are the smallest subdivisions in the lungs.
Muc	Muc(o)	O	Mucus	An important fluid substance that protects the lungs from going

				dry. And also trap some foreign particles like dust or bacteria.
Nas	Nas(o)	O	Nasal	Just in the case of the nasal cavity, where the first process of breathing occurs.
Ox	Ox(o)	O	Oxygen	Oxygen: an important element that is breathed in the body.

Pharyng	Pharyng(o)	O	Pharynx	The next respiratory organ after the nasal cavity.
Pleur	Pleur(o)	O	Pleura	An important part of the lungs that helps reduce friction between the lungs, the chest cavity, and the ribcage.
Pneum	Pneum(o)	O	Lungs or air	In the case of pneumonia or pneumothor

				ax, inflammation of the air sacs with fluid and leakage of air into the lungs space or the chest wall, respectively.
Pulmon	Pulmon(o)	O	Lungs	For example, pulmonary hypertension; a type of high blood pressure that affects the arteries of the lungs

				and the right side of the heart.
Ptysis		O	To split	For example, pyoptysis, which means separation of the pus.
Sinus '	Sinus(o)	O	Sinuses	In the case of sinusitis; inflammatio n of the cavities around the nasal passages.

Spir	Spir(o)	O	To breath	Like a spirometer, an apparatus used to measure the volume of air breathed in or out.
Tonsill	Tonsill(o)	O	Tonsil	In the case of tonsillitis, which is an inflammatio n of the tonsils.
Trache	Trache(o)	O	The trachea, also known as the	The trachea is a passage for oxygen to the lungs.

			windpipe	

Common disease terms associated with the Respiratory System.

Below are some common diseases associated with the respiratory system and their pharmacological treatment.

Asthma is a condition characterized by inflammation of the airways. The most effective drugs for this condition are Adrenoceptor agonists and glucocorticoids.

Chronic Obstructive Pulmonary Disease: This condition is characterized by lung disease that blocks airflow by making it difficult to breathe. The most common condition that makes up this condition is emphysema which chronic bronchitis. Bronchodilators and anticholinergics are used to treat this; they include salbutamol and terbutaline, then ipratropium and oxitropium, respectively.

Chronic Bronchitis: This is a common disease among smokers; a long-term bronchi inflammation characterizes it. It can be treated by using roflumilast, a phosphodiesterase-4 inhibitor.

Cystic Fibrosis: This is a life-threatening inherited disorder characterized by damage to the lungs and digestive system. This condition does not have a cure, but some drugs can ease the symptoms.

Emphysema: This is a condition characterized by damage to the alveoli in the lungs. It can be treated with corticosteroids like budesonide.

Lung Cancer: This happens mostly in people that smoke. It is a type of cancer that begins in the lungs and can be caused by smoking, family history, or exposure to harmful chemicals or toxins. The common pharmacological treatment for this includes drugs like carboplatin and cisplatin.

Pneumonia: Filling of fluid in the air sacs that causes inflammation. It can be treated by using antibiotics or vaccines.

Pleural Effusion: A condition characterized by a liquid in the tissue lining of the lungs and chest. Treatment can be done by removing the fluid or giving antibiotics.

Medical Terminologies According to The Circulatory System

Previously, you learned about breathing, intake of oxygen, and release of carbon dioxide, but where is that oxygen taken from the lungs? This is the role of the circulatory system. A healthy circulatory system is important in every human's life; it becomes life-threatening when it fails to deliver enough oxygen and nutrients. You will now take the journey of learning some exciting terminologies of the circulatory system, disease, and the little treatment will keep you wondering and thinking about how easy they are. The circulatory system is also known as the cardiovascular system. It comprises the heart and blood vessels. The primary function of this system is to deliver oxygen and other nutrients to the body and remove the waste products of metabolism. And this process is done by the network of blood vessels present in the heart. Along with the heart, three other systems also function in systemic circulation that you will see later.

There are three main circulations in the circulatory system:

The Pulmonary Circulation

In this type of circulation, blood moves between the heart and the lungs. It transports blood not combined with oxygen to the lungs to absorb oxygen and release carbon dioxide. Now the blood is mixed with oxygen, and it will then flow back to the heart.

The Systemic Circulation

From the heart, the systemic circulation will transport the blood to the other part of the body.

The Coronary Circulation

This is also part of the systemic circulation; the primary purpose of coronary circulation is to drain blood from the tissues of the heart.

The Heart

The heart is a muscular organ that pumps blood located in the mediastinum between the two lungs. The heart contains four chambers: the right atrium, right ventricle, left atrium, and left ventricle.

Vessels of The Heart

The main vessels in the heart are the superior vena cava, inferior veins cava, aorta, right coronary artery, left coronary artery, pulmonary artery, pulmonary vein, circumflex artery, and left anterior descending artery.

Below are the Medical Terminologies According to the Circulatory System

Terminologies	Combining Form	Vowel	Meaning	Example
Aden	Aden(o)	O	Gland	Like in the case of adenocarcinoma, a condition characterized by cancer development in the glands that line the organs.

Angi	Angi(o)	O	Vessel	For angiogenesis, a situation where new blood vessels are formed.
Aort	Aort(o)	O	Aorta	For example, the aorta; the largest artery in the body.
Arteri	Arteri(o)	O	Artery	The arteries that deliver oxygen combine with blood from the heart to the body tissues.
Ather	Ather(o)	O	Fatty	Fatty plague occurs when there is a

			plague	plague in the arteries, which can cause a reduction in blood flow.
Atri	Atri(o)	O	Atrium	The first to receive oxygenated blood from systemic circulation.
Cardi	Cardi(o)	O	Heart	In the case of cardiology which is the study of the heart.
Erythr	Erythr(o)	O	Red	For example, erythromycin, a medication used to treat a

				variety of bacterial infections.
Hem	Hem(o)	O	Blood	In the case of hemophilia, a disorder that occurs when the blood doesn't clot, typically resulting in excessive bleeding.
Hemat	Hemat(o)	O	Blood	Example Hematology; study of blood.
Leuc	Leuk(o)	O	White	For example, leukocytes are also called white blood

				cells that protect the body against bacteria and infection.
Lymph	Lymph(o)	O	Lymph	For example, lymphocytes are a type of white blood cell that defends the immune system against invading bacteria and infections.
Phleb	Phleb(o)	O	Vein	Phlebotomy: a situation where a needle is used to collect blood

				from the vein.
Splen	Splen(o)	O	Spleen	For example, splenomegaly, a condition characterized by enlargement of the spleen.
Thromb	Thromb(o)	O	Clot	Thrombosis: a condition when blood clots block the blood vessels.
Ven	Ven(o)	O	Vein	For example, the venous system, a network of veins that help deliver oxygenated

				blood back to the heart.
Ventricul	Ventricul(o)	O	Ventricle	For example, ventriculomegaly: condition characterized by prenatal ultrasound.

Common diseases terms associated with the circulatory system and some pharmacological treatments.

The circulatory system is prone to some diseases that can be mild, moderate, or even severe. They include:

Angina Pectoris: a condition characterized by reduced blood flow to the heart and can be treated by beta-blockers, calcium channel blockers, or nitrates.

Arrhythmia: when the heart's beating changes to either irregular, too fast, or too slow, the condition is termed arrhythmia, and it happens when the electrical impulses in the heart stop working properly. It can be treated by using beta-blockers, calcium channel blockers, or dietary supplements.

Atherosclerosis: when there is fat, cholesterol or other substances buildup in the artery's walls, the condition is termed atherosclerosis. It can be treated by using anticoagulant or cholesterol medications. Sometimes healthy diet and exercise will be of benefit in this condition.

Cardiac Ischemia: this is a condition characterized by a reduction in the cardiac muscle's ability to pump blood. Treatment depends on the severity of the condition. It can be treated by using angiotensin-converting enzymes, angiotensin receptor blockers, or anti-ischemic agents

Dysrhythmia: when there is an abnormal physiological rhythm in the activity of the brain or heart. The condition is called dysrhythmia. The pharmacological treatment for this condition is beta-blockers or calcium channel blockers

Heart Attack: when blood flow fails to reach the heart muscle due to the blockage, there is a reaction known as heart attack, which is life-threatening (also called myocardial infarction). The pharmacological treatment includes using anticoagulants, beta-blockers, or antianginal.

Heart Failure: when the heart fails to pump blood the way it is supposed to, a condition termed heart failure occurs. The pharmacological treatment includes using drug beta-blockers, diuretics, or dietary supplements.

High Blood Pressure: also called hypertension. It occurs when there is an increase in the force of blood against the wall of the arteries. Treatment includes using antihypertensive medications, beta-blockers, calcium channel blockers, or diuretics.

High Cholesterol: this is a condition characterized by increased cholesterol levels in the blood, decreasing blood flow and increasing the risk of heart attack and stroke. Medications include cholesterol medications, statin, healthy diets, and exercise.

Stroke: This is an emergency condition when there is obstruction or damage to the blood supplies to the brain. The pharmacological treatment includes using anticoagulants, an antihypertensive drug, ACE inhibitors, or alteplase.

Quick Exercises 9

Integumentary System

1. The _______ is the largest system in the body.

A. Skin B. Hair C. Stomach D. Heart

2. _______ is the first layer of the skin.

A. Dermis B. Epidermis C. Connective tissues D. Epithelium

Respiratory System

3. _________ is taken into the body during respiration and _________ is excreted from the body.

4. The first process of breathing occurs in the _________.

A. Mouth B. Lungs C. Nose D. Ear

Circulatory System

5. The heart is a muscular organ that consists of __________ chambers.

A. 1 B. 2 C. 3 D. 4

6. ___________ is the main purpose of coronary circulation.

Medical Terminologies According to The Digestive System

Whenever the digestive system is mentioned, the first thing that comes to mind is food. The digestive system is also called the gastrointestinal tract and the other accessory organs of digestion. Digestion is the breakdown of food into small components of easy absorption and assimilation. Many organs make up the digestive system. They are:

The Mouth

Where the first process of mechanical digestion occurs, the mouth breaks down the food particles by chewing. The salivary gland in the mouth secretes saliva, which moisture the food substances for easy swallowing.

The Pharynx

From the mouth, the food particles move to the pharynx, where it is swallowed.

The Esophagus

From the pharynx, the food substances are moved to the esophagus. The food substance here move in a peristalsis manner to the next organ of digestion.

The Stomach

Here, the food is mixed and grounded. The stomach secretes acid and enzymes that help in the further breakdown of food particles, changing it from solid form to liquid or paste.

The Small Intestine

The small intestine absorbs all the food nutrients. Food substance from the stomach enters the small intestine, where the nutrients are absorbed. After that, it is moved to the next organ of digestion.

The Large Intestine

The food substances are then moved to the large intestine, where salt and water are absorbed from the remaining undigested foods. From here, the waste product is then transferred to the next organ of digestion.

The Rectum

The rectum stores the waste product of digestion until there is a need for evacuation.

The Anus

This is where the digestion process ends. The waste product of digestion is removed from the body through the anus.

Terminologies	Combining Form	Vowel	Meaning	Example
Abdomin	Abdomin (o)	O	Abdomen	Abdominocentesis; a process in which a needle is used surgically to extract fluid from the stomach.
Aden	Aden(o)	O	Gland	Adenocarcinoma colon: deadly cancerous cells developed in

				the rectum and colon.
Aliment	Aliment(o)	O	Food	Alimento: known as food, any substance that is consumed to provide nutritional value to the body.
Amyl	Amyl(o)	O	Starch	In the case of amyloid: abnormal development of protein deposited in some organs or tissue of the body.

An	An(o)	O	Anus	Ano-fistula: a condition characterized by an infected tunnel between skin and the anus.
Append	Append(o)	O	Appendix	Example: appendectomy: surgical removal of the appendix after getting infected.
Ase			Enzyme	For example: the enzyme Amylase helps in the digestion of food.

Bucc	Bucc(o)	O	Cheek	Like buccopharyngeal: a site near the cheek and the pharynx.
Cec	Cec(o)	O	Cecum	Example: cecostomy: a procedure done in children to remove feces when other treatments fail to work.
Cheil	Cheil(o)	O	Lips	Like Cheilosis: when the corners of the mouth get inflamed or an appearance of

				small cracks, the condition is termed cheilosis.
Cholecyst	Cholecyst (o)	O	Gallbladder	Cholecystostomy: a procedure that involves the placement of a drainage catheter in the gall bladder.
Choled	Choled(o)	O	Common bile duct	In the case of choledochotomy, the procedure is done in patients with cholelithiasis, a surgical incision of the

				common bile duct.
Col	Col(o)	O	Colon	Colorectal polyp, which is formed on the colon and rectal.
Dent	Dent(o)	O	Tooth	Like the Dentoalveolar abscess, which is when an infection causes a pus pocket in the tooth.
Duoden	Duoden (o)	O	Duodenu m	For example, Duodenoscope , an instrument used to see the

				small intestine.
Enter	Enter(o)	O	Small Intestine	In the case of Enterotomy, a surgical incision into the intestine.
Epiglott			Epiglottis	For example: the epiglottis is a cartilage situated in the throat, behind the trachea, and in front of the larynx.
Esophag	Esophag(o)	O	Esophagus	For example, Esophagectomy, a surgical procedure, is done to treat esophageal

				cancer.
Gastr	Gastr(o)	O	Stomach	The gastrointestinal tract, which is the alimentary canal or the digestive tract.
Gloss	Gloss(o)	O	Tongue	For example, the glossopharyngeal nerve.
Hepat	Hepat(o)	O	Liver	For example, the hepatocytes are the chief functional cells of the

				liver.
Ile	Ile(o)	O	Ileum	For example, an ileostomy; a surgical opening in the abdominal wall.
Intestin	Intestin(o)	O	Intestine	For example, the intestino-intestinal inhibitory reflex, which is the effect of distension on intestinal slow waves.
Jejun	Jejun(o)	O	Jejunum	Jejunostomy is a procedure done to administer

				nutrition in the lumen of the proximal jejunum.
Lith	Lith(o)	O	Stone, calculus	For example, lithotomy, a surgical procedure done to remove calculus inside organs.
Or	Or(o)	O	Mouth	The oropharynx, which is the middle part of the pharynx situated behind the oral cavity.

Pancreat	Pancreat(o)	O	Pancreas	In the case of pancreatectomy, the surgical removal of some portion of the pancreas.
Periton	Periton(o)	O	Peritoneum	For example, peritonitis, which is a situation whereby the lining of the abdominal walls gets inflamed.
Pharyng	Pharyng(o)	O	Pharynx	For example, pharyngotonsillitis, the inflammation of the pharynx

				and the tonsils.
Proct	Proct(o)	O	Rectum	For example, proctocolitis, a term used to describe rectum or colon inflammation.
Sial	Sial(o)	O	Saliva	For example, maple, Sialosis, a condition characterized by swelling of the salivary gland.
Sigmoid	Sigmoid(o)	O	Sigmoid colon	For example, Sigmoidoscopy, the clinical examination of

				the rectum and the sigmoid colon.

Some diseases associated with the Digestive System and their Pharmacological treatment

There are many diseases associated with the digestive system; they all Fissure: this is a condition characterized by a tunnel between the anus and the skin. It can be treated with surgery — Fistulotomy.

Celiac Disease: a condition characterized by an immune reaction to eaten gluten. It can be treated by eating a gluten-free diet and dietary supplements or vitamins.

Crohn's Disease: also known as ileitis, is a bowel disease in which the lining of the digestive tract gets inflamed. It can be treated with an anti-inflammatory drug, non-steroidal anti-inflammatory drug, or vitamins.

Diverticulitis: This disease commonly occurs in people from the age of 40; it's characterized by small pouches, inflammation, or infection in the gastrointestinal tract. It can be treated with antibiotics or dietary supplements.

Gallstones: a condition characterized by a hard deposit in the fluid inside the gallbladder. It can be treated with surgery called cholecystectomy or by taking cholesterol medications or eating a low-fat diet.

Hemorrhoids: also known as piles, are characterized by inflammation of veins in the rectum and anus, causing bleeding and discomfort. It can be treated with dietary supplements or local anesthetics.

Irritable Bowel Syndrome: when there is pain in the intestine accompanied by diarrhea and constipation, the condition is termed irritable bowel syndrome. The pharmacological treatment includes antibiotics, anti-diarrhea, dietary supplements, or laxatives.

Medical Terminologies According to The Reproductive System

The continuous production of organisms that is from the same species is known as reproduction. The reproductive system is vital in keeping a species alive. It consists of the organs that are responsible for the production of offspring. In general, reproduction is when a male sexual cell is deposited into the female sexual organ, which gets fertilized and leads to the production of a fetus.

The reproductive system is divided into two:

The Female Reproductive System

The female reproductive system plays an essential role in reproduction; it consists of organs that produce a new individual.

Below are the organs and functions of the female reproductive system:

Ovaries: the ovaries play an important role in producing the egg cells called ova or oocytes, transported to the fallopian tube where they wait for sperm for fertilization.

When the egg gets fertilized, it's then transported to the uterus, where it gets implanted into the thick uterine lining and continues developing. In the uterus, if fertilization does not occur, the uterine wall sheds, producing blood called menstruation.

The female reproductive system also produces some hormones. The production of these hormones and menstruation stops when a woman reaches a stage called menopause.

Anatomical Makeup of The Female Reproductive System

The female reproductive system consists of external and internal structures:

External Structures

Labia majora: this is the first external feature of the female reproductive system, which protects the internal organs.

Labia minora: beneath the labia majora is the labia minora surrounding the vaginal opening and the urethra.

Bartholin's glands: These glands produce mucus secretion, and they are located on each side next to the vaginal opening.

Clitoris: is situated at the midpoint of the two labia minora. This is a sensitive area that is comparable to the male penis.

Vagina: the vagina joins the cervix to the outer body. It is also called the birth canal.

The uterus: also called the womb, is a hollow, pear-shaped organ that houses a fetus. It is divided into two parts; the cervix and the corpus.

Hormones that a role in the female reproductive system include:

- Follicle-stimulating hormone
- Luteinizing hormone
- Estrogen
- Progesterone

The woman's reproductive system consists of about 7-8million eggs.

The Male Reproductive System

The Male reproductive system functions in maintaining and transporting sperm and semen into the female reproductive tract during intercourse.

Many hormones are responsible for the process of reproduction in males, including:

- Testosterone
- Follicle-stimulating hormone
- Luteinizing hormone

The male reproductive system consists of many organs that function in human reproduction, including:

The penis that functions in sexual intercourse with an opening that delivers sperm cells into the female genitalia.

The scrotum is a punch sac situated beneath the penis and contains the testes.

The testes are responsible for the production of testosterone which leads to the production of sperm cells.

The epididymis stores and transports the sperm cell after they are produced in the testes.

Vas deferens transports mature cells to the urethra.

Ejaculatory ducts are emptied into the urethra.

The urethra function in the ejaculation of semen when the male reaches orgasm.

Seminal vesicles supply the sperm with fructose which provides energy that helps the sperm cells to move.

The prostate glands produce fluids that help in nourishing the sperm cells.

The bulbourethral gland produces liquid that lubricates the urethra.

Below are medical terminologies according to the reproductive system.

Terminologies	Combining form	Vowel	Meaning
Amni	Amni(o)	O	Amnion
Cervic	Cervic(o)	O	Cervix of the uterus
Colp	Colp(o)	O	Vagina
Embry	Embry(o)	O	Embryo
Gravida	Gravida(o)	O	Pregnancy
Gyn	Gyn(o)	O	Female
Hyster	Hyster(o)	O	Uterus

Lact	Lact(o)	O	Milk
Mamm	Mamm(o)	O	Breast
Men	Men(o)	O	Menstruation
Nat	Nat(o)	O	Birth
Oophoro	Oophoro(o)	O	Ovary
Orch	Orch(o)	O	Testes
Ov	Ov(o)	O	Egg
Salping	Salping(o)	O	Fallopian tube
Sperm	Sperm(o)	O	Sperm
Spermat	Spermat(o)	O	Sperm

Common conditions associated with the reproductive system with their pharmacological treatment

Uterine fibroids: this affects women during their childbearing years. It's a developing non-cancerous growth and can be treated with hormones or sex hormone suppression medications.

Sexually transmitted diseases (STDs): this is an infection that is transmitted during sexual intercourse, and they are of many types, including; genital herpes, human papillomavirus, chlamydia, etc. The treatment depends on the cause of the illness.

Testicular cancer: when cancer affects the testicles, the condition is called testicular cancer. It can be treated with chemotherapy or surgery.

Infertility: This is a situation characterized by failure to get pregnant after multiple unprotected sexual for a year. Although some causes of Infertility might not be known, the treatment always depends on the grounds of infertility.

Medical Terminologies According to The Nervous System

The nervous system is often called the command center in the human body. The nervous system originates from the brain and controls almost all activities of the body. The nervous system has many functions.

Below are a few functions of the nervous system:

- Maintenance of Homeostasis
- Memory and Learning
- Programming of the Spinal Cord
- Control of Voluntary Movement

The nervous system is divided into two:

The Central Nervous System (CNS)

The central nervous system consists of the brain and the spinal cord. They work in integrating information received from the peripheral nervous systems and also function in decision making. The CNS is the head office of the body because it is designed to control all actions in the body voluntarily and involuntarily.

The Peripheral Nervous System (PNS)

The peripheral nervous system consists of the cranial nerves and the spinal nerves. They send and receive information between the central nervous system and the rest of the body.

Further Division of the Nervous System

The nervous system is further divided into the following divisions.

The sensory division carries impulses from outside the body to the CNS and PNS, e.g., touching, hearing, sight, etc.

The motor division transfers impulses to different parts of the body like the glands, muscles, and organs from the CNS and PNS.

The Somatic Nervous System

This part of the nervous system is also called voluntary division. They are nerves that end in the skeletal muscles. They transfer impulses that control the skeletal muscles when they receive an order from the brain.

The Autonomic Nervous System conducts impulses to the internal organs or viscera. E.g., the lungs, GIT, and glands.

There is the sympathetic division that works to mobilize the body during fight or flight response.

The parasympathetic division that got activated when the body is at rest and enhances digestion.

Brain

The brain is part of the nervous system that is responsible for making decisions and processing information. And it is always on standby. The brain consists of the cerebrum, hypothalamus, corpus collusion, ventricles, thalamus, midbrain, cerebellum, brain stem, pituitary gland, pons, and medulla.

Spinal Cord

The spinal cord can be likened to a road through which information from receptors travels to the brain and from the brain to the remaining part of the body.

Below is a Table of Medical Terminologies according to the Nervous system

Terminologies	Combining Form	Vowel	Meaning
Algesi	Algesi(o)	O	Excessive

			sensitivity to pain
Cerebel	Cerebel(o)	O	Cerebellum
Cerebr	Cerebr(o)	O	Cerebrum
Electr	Electr(o)	O	Electricity
Enchephal	Enchephal(o)	O	Brain
Mening	Mening(o)	O	Meninges
Ment	Ment(o)	O	Mind
Myel	Myel(o)	O	Spinal cord
My	My(o)	O	Muscle
Neur	Neur(o)	O	Nerve

Phas	Phas(o)	O	Speech
Pont	Pont(o)	O	Pons
Psych	Psych (o)	O	Mind
Redicul	Redicul(o)	O	Nerve root
Thalam	Thalam(o)	O	Thalamus
Ventricul	Ventricul(o)	O	Ventricles

Common Conditions Associated with the Nervous System and their Pharmacological Treatment

The conditions that affect the nervous system also affect the rest of the body because it controls almost all body activities.

Below are some disorders that can affect the nervous system with a simple solution to solve the problem.

Alzheimer's Disease: a disease that progresses to destroy memory and other vital functions in the brain. The condition can be treated with cognition-enhancing medications.

Amnesia: occurs when the brain gets injured caused by trauma, illness, alcohol, or drugs, resulting in an inability to remember things that happened for a time.

Bell's Palsy: also known as idiopathic facial paralysis. A condition characterized by weakening in the half-face muscles. Treatment can be done with antiviral drugs.

Cerebral Palsy: a condition in which there is a congenital disorder in movement and the muscle or posture. It can be treated with sedatives or muscle relaxants. In some aspects, exercise can also be of help.

Dementia: This is a condition characterized by loss of memory or thinking ability. It can be managed with cognitive-enhancing medication. Sometimes rehabilitation and therapy might help.

Insomnia: a condition characterized by problems in falling asleep or staying asleep. Medications include antihistamines, antidepressants, and sedatives.

Epilepsy: a seizure disorder caused by a disturbance in the nerve cell activity in the brain. It can be treated with anticonvulsants, nerve pain medication, or sedatives.

Motor Neurone Disease (MND): is a disorder that affects the brain and nerves. The sad thing about MND is, it has no cure, but treatment and medications can help to control some of the symptoms.

Multiple Sclerosis: is a disease that causes nerve damage resulting in obstruction in the brain and body communication. It can be treated with anti-inflammatory, chemotherapy, or steroids.

Parkinson's Disease: this is a disorder that affects movement. It can be treated with antidepressants, anti-tremor, cognitive-enhancing medications, or dopamine promoters.

Sciatica: a pain that affects the legs and the lower back caused by herniated disc or bone spur. Although treatment depends on the severity, it can be treated with analgesics, muscle relaxants, nonsteroidal anti-inflammatory drugs, or nerve pain medication.

Quick Exercise 10

Digestive System

1. _________ is a condition characterized by inflammation of veins in the rectum and anus, causing bleeding and discomfort.

A. Sciatica B. Hemorrhoid C. Acne D. Celiac disease

2. ___________ is a disease that commonly occurs in people from the age of 40 and is characterized by small pouches inflammation or infection in the gastrointestinal tract.

A. Diverticulitis B. Parkinson's disease C. Hemorrhoid D. Crohn's disease

Reproductive System

3. __________is situated at the midpoint of the two labia minora.

A. Labia majora B. Labia minora C. Clitoris D. Fallopian tubes

4. _________ is not part of the male reproductive system.

A. Penis B. Testes C. Uterus D. Scrotum

Nervous System

5. List the four functions of the nervous system.

6. _________ is a disease that progresses and destroys memory and other important function in the brain.

A. Parkinson's disease B. Multiple Sclerosis C. Alzheimer's disease D. Cerebral palsy

Medical Terminologies According to The Lymphatic System

The lymphatic system is one of the major parts of the immune system with many important functions:

- It protects the body from illness caused by invaders.
- It maintains the level of the body fluid.
- It absorbs fat from the digestive tracts.
- It removes cellular waste products.

The lymphatic system is part of the immune system that consists of tissue networks, vessels, and organs that act together to return the lymph to the circulatory system. The lymph is a colorless and watery fluid that is moved back to the bloodstream.

The lymphatic system consists of the following parts:

Lymph: also known as lymphatic fluid. Extra fluid is collected from the cell, tissues, and other substances. The lymph also contains and transports lymphocytes to their site of action.

Lymph Nodes: they are bean-shaped glands that help monitor and cleanse the lymph as it passes through them.

They clear out cancer and damaged cells. There are about 600lymph nodes inside the body. Some are single existence, while others exist as groups connected by lymphatic vessels. Some of the familiar locations of the lymph nodes include the neck, armpit, and Lymphatic Vessels: they are vessels that help in transporting the lymph away from the tissues.

Collecting Ducts: after collecting fluids from the tissues and organs, it is emptied into a collecting duct or thoracic duct, which helps return lymph to the circulatory system. This collecting duct also prevents edema.

Spleen: also called the blood bank of the body, helps filter and store blood cells that fight invading diseases or bacteria.

Thymus: it helps it mature the specific cells that help fight foreign organisms.

Tonsils and adenoids: these part of the lymphatic system helps in trapping pathogens from food or air. They are termed the body's first line of defense against foreign invaders.

Bone Marrow: soft tissues enter some bones like breast and hip bone that houses red blood cells, white blood cells, and platelets.

Peyer's Patches: they are masses of lymphoid tissues present in the mucous membrane that lines the small intestine and destroys bacteria.

Appendix: the appendix houses good bacteria and helps in destroying harmful bacteria before they reach the intestine. Disease or infection can affect the functions of the lymphatic system.

Terminologies	Combining Form	Vowel	Meaning
Aden	Aden(o)	O	Gland
Bas	Bas(o)	O	Base
Eosin	Eosin(o)	O	Red or rosy

Erythr	Erythr(o)	O	Red
Granul	Granul(o)	O	Granules
Hem	Hem(o)	O	Blood
Hemat	Hemat(o)	O	Blood
Immun	Immun(o)	O	Protection
Kary	Kary(o)	O	Nucleus
Leuk	Leuk(o)	O	White
Lymph	Lymph(o)	O	Lymph
Lymphangi	Lymphagi(o)	O	Lymph gland
Mon	Mon(o)	O	One or single

Morpho	Morpho(o)	O	Shape
Myel	Myel(o)	O	Bone marrow
Necr	Necr(o)	O	Death
Neutr	Neutr(o)	O	Neither
Nucle	Nucle(o)	O	Nucleus
Phleb	Phleb(o)	O	Vein
Sider	Sider(o)	O	Iron
Spher	Spher(o)	O	Globe
Splen	Splen(o)	O	Spleen
Thromb	Thromb(o)	O	Clot

Thym	Thym(o)	O	Thymus
Tonsil	Tonsil (o)	O	Tonsil

Common Conditions Associated with The Lymphatic System

Common disorders associated with the lymphatic system include:

Lymphoma: this disease is of two types, Hodgkin's Lymphoma and non-Hodgkin's Lymphoma: lymphoma is the cancer of the lymphatic system. It can be treated with bone marrow therapy, radiation therapy, and chemotherapy.

Lymphangitis: they are swollen lymph nodes; enlarge the immune system in response to bacterial or viral infection.

Lymphadenitis: a condition characterized by inflammation of the lymph nodes.

Lymphedema: when there is an obstruction in the flow of lymph causing arm or leg swelling. The condition is termed lymphedema. The treatment involves exercise and using moisturizers.

Lymphocytosis: this is a harmless and temporary condition but can sometimes represent a serious issue. It occurs when your immune system is working to defend your body against disease and infection. An increase in white blood cells characterizes it.

Medical Terminologies According to The Endocrine System

The endocrine system connects glands that work to make the hormone that helps in cell communication. This system is responsible for the majority of the cell and organs functioning in the body.

Gland

To gland is an organ that produces hormones that work in the body.

Functions of the endocrine system include:

Producing hormones that control activities in the body, such as growth, metabolism, and reproduction.

Regulate how the hormones are being released.

Transport the hormones to the blood, where they are taken to their site of action.

Parts of the Endocrine System

Many glands come together to form the endocrine system. They include:

The Hypothalamus: hypothalamus connects the brain with the endocrine system.

The pituitary Gland: is also called the master gland because it regulates almost all the activities of the other glands. It is divided into two anterior pituitary glands that secret six hormones; growth hormone follicle-stimulating hormone, luteinizing hormone, prolactin, thyroid hormone, adrenocorticotropic hormone, and the posterior pituitary gland that secrete two hormones; antidiuretic hormone and oxytocin.

Pineal Gland: it secretes the hormone melatonin.

Thyroid Gland: it secretes the thyroid hormones, which are triiodothyronine, tetraiodothyronine, and calcitonin.

Parathyroid gland: it secretes the hormone parathyroid hormone.

Thymus: it secretes the t-cells of white blood cells and fights against bacteria. It is also important in child development.

Adrenal Gland: the adrenal gland is divided into two, the adrenal cortex and the adrenal medical. They secrete the hormones corticosteroids.

Pancreas: the pancreas produces digestive ensures that aid in digestion in the gastrointestinal tract.

Ovaries: the ovaries produce estrogen and progesterone that function during puberty, regulate the menstrual cycle and help during pregnancy.

Testes: the testes produce testosterone that helps in male growth.

Below are Medical Terminologies According to the Endocrine System.

Terminologies	Combining form	Vowel	Meaning
Gluc	Gluc(o)	O	Sugar or sweet
Oid			Resembling

Ose			Sugar
Parathyroid	Parathyroid(o)	O	Parathyroid glands
Thym	Thym(o)	O	Thymus gland
Thyr	Thyr(o)	O	Thyroid gland
Toxic	Toxic(o)	O	Toxin

Common disorders associated with the endocrine system with their pharmacological treatment

When the endocrine system is not working properly, there will be a severe problem in development from many aspects, including pregnancy, puberty, weight gain and loss, energy, sugar, etc.

Below are some disorders associated with the endocrine system, with a solution to each.

Acromegaly: This disorder is characterized by excess secretion of growth hormone in adults by the pituitary gland. The pharmacological treatment includes administering synthetic hormones and dopamine promoters.

Addison's disease: when the adrenal gland fails to produce adequate hormones, this disorder is termed Addison's Disease. It can be treated by administering steroids medications.

Cushing's syndrome: when a patient is exposed to high cortisol levels for a while, it results in a disorder called Cushing's Syndrome. It can be treated by reducing steroid use, surgery, or radiation.

Diabetes mellitus: this is a condition characterized by an increase in blood sugar level leading to damage to the heart and blood vessels. Treatments include adapting to a healthy diet and insulin medications.

Graves disease: this condition mainly affects women from 40; a butterfly-shaped gland in the throat characterizes it. Treatment includes the administration of beta-blockers or anti-thyroid agents.

Hashimoto's thyroiditis: this is related to graves disease; it occurs when the butterfly-shaped gland got attacked by the immune system. It can be treated with synthetic hormone medication.

Hyperthyroidism: This disorder occurs when there is excess secretion of the thyroid hormones. It can be treated with beta-blocker and antithyroid agent medications.

Hypothyroidism: this condition is characterized by a reduction in the normal secretion of the thyroid hormones. It can be treated with thyroid hormone replacement.

Prolactinoma: this is characterized by a tumor in the pituitary gland. It can be treated with a dopamine promoter, surgery, or radiation.

Medical Terminologies According to The Urinary System

After eating and drinking, the body absorbs the valuable nutrients and aliments the useless ones. And this is where the urinary system plays its vital role. The urinary system keeps the body in balance by excreting all the unwanted substances, including urea, extra salt, and extra water.

Parts and functions of the urinary system

The urinary system consists of several parts and functions, including:

Kidneys: these are bean-shaped pairs of organs that function in removing from the blood and transporting it out of the body in the form of urine.

Ureters: the functions of this organ in transporting the urine from the kidneys to the bladder.

Bladder: this function in storing urine until the need for voiding arises.

Urethra: This is an organ that allows urine to move out of the body.

Below are some medical terminologies associated with the urinary system.

Terminologies	Combining form	Vowel	Meaning
Bacteri	Bacteri(o)	O	Bacteria
Cyst	Cyst(o)	O	Bladder or sac

Glumerul	Glumerul(o)	O	Glomerulus
Hemat	Hemat(o)	O	Blood
Lith	Lith(o)	O	Stone or calculus
Nephr	Nephr(o)	O	Nephron
Noct	Noct(o)	O	Night
Py	Py(o)	O	Pus
Pyel	Pyel(o)	O	Renal pelvis
Ur	Ur(o)	O	Urine
Ureter	Ureter(o)	O	Ureter
Urethr	Urethr(o)	O	Urethra

Ren	Ren(o)	O	Nephron

Common disorders associated with the urinary system

Urinary tract infection: this is a disease that mostly occurs in females but also occurs in males; it affects the urinary system like the bladder and the urethra, and when it gets serious, it affects the kidneys. It can be treated with antibiotics

Incontinence: this is a condition characterized by a lack of voluntary control over urination. Most treatment involves medications and psychotherapy.

Kidney disease: this is a life-threatening disorder that results in kidney failure. It occurs when the kidney fails to excrete waste products. Treatment includes peritoneal dialysis, hemofiltration, or dialysis.

Kidney stones: there are small hard substances formed in the kidney, which is sometimes painful. Treatment includes medications like narcotics, non-steroidal anti-inflammatory drugs, or diuretics.

Quick Exercise 11

Lymphatic System

1. ________ is known as the blood bank in the body.

   A. Thymus B. Spleen C. Thyroid Gland D. Heart

2. When there is an obstruction in the flow of lymph, causing arm or leg swelling. The condition is termed __________.

   A. Lymphedema B. Parkinson's disease C. Cushing's syndrome D. Lymph nodes

Endocrine System

3. The pituitary gland is divided into ________ categories.

4. Excess secretion of growth hormone in adults leads to ________.

Urinary System

5. _________function in storing urine until the need for voiding arises.

A. Bladder B. Ureter C. Kidney D. Penis

6. __________ is an organ that allows urine to move out of the body.

A. Urethra B. Ureter C. Kidney D. Fallopian tube

Medical Terminologies According to The Musculoskeletal System

The musculoskeletal system is the body that aids the body in movement, shape, support, and stability. The musculoskeletal system is divided into two (2) broad systems:

1. The muscular system consists of all the different types of muscles and tendons.
2. The skeletal system consists of the bones, cartilage, and joints.

Functions Of the Musculoskeletal System

- It gives the body shape and stability.
- The skeletal system protects the vital organs in the body like the lungs, heart, and brain.
- The muscular system plays a vital role in body heat production.
- The skeletal system serves as storage for minerals like calcium.
- The muscular system consists of specialized muscle tissue. The muscle tissues are divided into three;

- A cardiac muscle that forms the musculature of the heart.
- Smooth muscles that overload vessels and hollow organs.
- Skeletal muscles are attached to the bones and help voluntary movements.

Under histological appearance, the cardiac and skeletal muscles are striated, while the smooth muscles are non-striated. The skeletal muscle is the only muscle that can be controlled because the somatic part of the nervous system innovates them. In contrast, the cardiac and smooth muscles are controlled involuntarily, so they are innovated by the autonomic nervous system.

The musculoskeletal system forms the functional unit of the muscular system. The human body consists of more than 600 muscles that vary in shape and size. The smallest muscle in the human body is the stapedius muscle located in the ear and the largest in the quadriceps femoral muscle located in the thigh.

The musculoskeletal system consists of four groups situated in all regions of the body.

Muscles Situated in The Head and Truck

These include the facial expressions muscles, mastication muscles, larynx and pharynx muscles, etc.

Muscles Situated in The Trunk

These include the back muscles, anterior and lateral abdominal muscles, and pelvis floor muscles.

Muscles Situated in The Upper Limbs

These include the shoulder muscles, arm muscles, forearm, and hand muscles.

Muscle Situated in The Lower Limbs

These include the muscles of the hip and thigh, muscles of the leg and foot also.

Skeletal muscles are composed of myocytes and muscular fibers.

The main physiological properties of the skeletal muscles include:

- Excitability is the ability to detect neural stimuli.
- Contractibility is the ability of the muscles to respond to neural stimuli.

- Extensibility allows the muscles to stretch without tearing.
- Elasticity allows the muscles to return to their original form after being extended.

Below are some of the movements that the musculoskeletal system performs:

- Flexion and extension
- Addiction and abduction
- Rotation
- Supination and pronation

The human skeleton consists of 206 bones associated with cartilage.

There are two divisions of the human bone:

- The axial skeleton
- The appendicular skeleton.

The bones are rigid structures that are made of calcified dense connective tissues. They are composed of a mineralized bone matrix consisting of type 1 collagen fiber. Each bone consists of two layers; compact bone and spongy bone.

There are different classes of bone according to shape, including:

- The long bone that is longitudinally long, e.g., humerus, ulna and tibia
- Short bone, e.g., the carpal bones
- Flat bones, e.g., the skull and sternum bone
- Sesamoid bones, e.g., the patella
- Irregular bones, e.g., the hip bone and the skull bones.

Cartilage

The cartilages are flexible connective tissues present in many organs of the body. It is composed of chondrocytes.

The cartilages are classified into many types, including:

- Hyaline cartilage
- Elastic cartilage
- Fibrocartilage
- Joints

A Joint is a place where two or more bones meet.

Joints are classified into:

- Synovial joints
- Fibrous joints
- Cartilaginous joints
- Ligaments

Ligaments are similar to tendons in structure. This connects bone to bone.

Tendons

They connect muscles to bone.

Terminologies	Combining form	Vowel	Meaning
Ankylos	Ankylos(o)	O	Stiffening
Arthr	Arthr(o)	O	Joint
Carp	Carp(o)	O	Wrist
Cervic	Cervic(o)	O	Neck

Chondr	Chondr(o)	O	Cartilage
Cost	Cost(o)	O	Ribs
Crani	Crani(o)	O	Skull
Dactyl	Dactyl(o)	O	Digit
Femor	Femor(o)	O	Thighbone
Fibul	Fibul(o)	O	Fibula
Humer	Humer(o)	O	Humerus
Ili	Ili(o)	O	Ileum
Lamin	Lamin(o)	O	Lamina of a vertebra

Mandibul	Mandibul(o)	O	Mandible
Maxill	Maxill(o)	O	Maxilla
Muscul	Muscul(o)	O	Muscle
Orth	Orth(o)	O	Straight
Oste	Oste(o)	O	Bone
Patell	Patell(o)	O	Kneecap
Pelvi	Pelv(i)	I	Pelvis
Phalang	Phalang(o)	O	Fingers or toes
Rachi	Rachi(o)	O	Vertebra
Vertebr	Vertebr(o)	O	Vertebra

Stern	Stern(o)	O	Sternum
Tend	Tend(o)	O	Tendon
Tibi	Tibi(o)	O	Tibia

Common disorders associated with the musculoskeletal system and their pharmacological treatment.

Arthritis: This condition worsens with age. It is characterized by inflammation of one or two joints that causes pain and stiffness. It can be treated with nonsteroidal anti-inflammatory drugs, analgesic, or narcotic medications.

Muscular dystrophy: this is a group of genetic diseases causing progressive weakness and loss of muscle mass. Treatment includes steroids and sometimes physical therapy.

Osteoporosis: this is a condition characterized by bone weakness and brittle. It can be treated with dietary supplements, vitamins, bone health, and hormone.

Sarcopenia: this condition is characterized by progressive and generalized loss of muscle mass and strength. It can be treated with constant physical exercise.

Medical Terminologies According to The Special Senses in The Body

The five special senses present in man are the:

- Smell
- Taste
- Sight
- Hearing
- Touch

Functions of the special senses include:

Vision: when a human is capable of seeing things around his surroundings. It's termed vision. This is achieved by the photoreceptors present in the retina. And this allows one to differentiate colors.

Hearing: The ability to perceive sound is also part of the special senses present in man.

Taste: when a human is capable of detecting the taste of substance by the tongue. This feature is termed taste sense.

Smell: the ability to perceive the odor of various features is called the sense of smell.

Touch: the touch receptors present in the skin allow sensing of touch.

The eye consists of 70% of the sensory receptors.

Anatomy Of Sensory Organs

For learning, vision is the most important feature needed. It's amazing when humans see what they are expected to see.

External and accessory structures of vision

Other accessory structures help in vision; they include:

- The eyelids that protect the eye.
- The eyelashes situated at the upper and lower border of the eyelids.
- Tarsal glands produce an oily secretion that lubricates the eye.
- Conjunctiva that lines the eyelids.
- Lacrimal apparatus that consists of the lacrimal glands.

- The lacrimal glands that secrete salt solution popularly known as tears.
- Lacrimal canaliculi: this is a passage for tears.
- Lysozyme: The lacrimal secretion contains antibodies and lysozymes that help in destroying bacteria and helps in cleaning the eyes, and also moistens and lubricates the eye.

The eyes also contain muscles including lateral rectus, medial rectus, inferior rectus, inferior oblique, and superior oblique.

The eye is spherical and hollow, with its walls having three layers, and the inside is filled, which helps keep the eye in shape called humor.

The layers that form the wall of the eyeballs include; the fibrous layer, Sclera, Cornea, vascular layer, Choroid, Ciliary body, Pupil, Sensory layer, Pigmented layer, Neutral layer, Two-neuron chain, Optic disc, Fovea centralis.

Lens: The lens makes the light entering the eye get focused on the retina. The eye lens divides the eye into two segments, the anterior segment that contains the clear watery fluid and the posterior segment, which contains a gel-like substance called the vitreous humor.

Eye Reflexes: These are reflexes necessary for the normal functioning of the eye.

Photopupillary Reflex: When bright light hits the eye, the pupils constrict immediately, which stops the excess light from causing harm to the photoreceptors. This is called the photopupillary reflex.

Accommodation Papillary Reflex: When a close object is viewed, the eye constricts to provide a better acute vision.

The Ear: The ear is the sense organ responsible for hearing and balance.

Anatomy of The Ear

The ear is anatomically divided into three major parts: the external, middle, and internal ear.

The External Ear: It is composed of the Auricle, the surface around the auditory canal opening. The External acoustic meets that secrete earwax to trap foreign bodies, and the Tympanic membrane, also called the eardrum.

Middle Ear: It is also called the tympanic cavity. It has an opening, a pharyngotympanic tube, and vesicles.

Internal Ear: It is a bony structure situated behind the eye socket deep in the temporal bone. It is also called the labyrinth. It is divided into three which are spiraling. The subdivisions are pea-sized cochlea, vestibule and semicircular canals.

The bony labyrinth has a plasma-like fluid-filled in it called perilymph, and suspended to it is the membranes labyrinth that follows the bony labyrinth. It contains endolymph. The endolymph is a thick fluid found in the membrane's labyrinth.

The Sense of Taste

The origin of taste comes from the Latin word "gustare," meaning to taste.

Taste Buds

Receptors of taste are vastly spread across the oral cavity and are mostly situated in the tongue.

The Papillae

The circumvallate and fungiform papillae

The glossopharyngeal nerve and the facial nerve supply the taste organs.

Mechanism of Hearing

The sound waves follow a route through the ear.

Vibrations

Sound waves vibrations pass through the air, membrane, fluid, and bone

The cochlea present in the ear helps transmit sound easier

When the frequency of the sound wave is low, it travels only around the cochlea, while the frequency of high sound waves passes through the cochlea.

The cochlea helps in transmitting sound waves in the ear.

Terminologies	Combining form	Vowel	Meaning
Audi	Audi(o)	O	Sound or hearing

Aur	Aur(o)	O	Ear
Blephar	Blephar(o)	O	Eyelid
Conjunctiva	Conjunctiva(o)	O	Conjunctivae
Corne	Corne(o)	O	Cornea
Myring	Myring(o)	O	Eardrum
Ocul	Ocul(o)	O	Eye
Olfact	Olfact(o)	O	Smell
Retin	Retin(o)	O	Retina

Common disorders associated with the special senses in man

Color blindness: This is a condition characterized by an inability to differentiate colors. Most of the time, this disorder is inherited. Although there is no cure for the condition, special glasses and contact lenses help a lot.

Deafness: A condition characterized by an inability to hear sound caused by inner ear nerve damage. It can be partial or complete deafness. Treatment depends on the severity of the illness. It can be treated with device therapy like a cochlear implant or bone-anchored hearing aid.

Anosmia: This condition is characterized by total inability to detect odor, it can be congenital, and treatment might be better by using antihistamines, nasal drops, or nasal steroids sprays.

Quick Exercise 12

Musculoskeletal System

1. _________ connects muscle to bone.

   A. Tendon B. Ligament C. Joint D. Skull

Special Senses

2. _________this is a condition characterized by inability to differentiate colors.

   A. Deafness B. Color blindness C. Parkinson's disease
D. Cushing's syndrome

3. List the five special senses in humans.

CONCLUSION

This book has been particularly helpful to you either as a medical student or an expert. You have been able to grasp how to memorize, retain, and recall words that have extended to medical terminologies. You can now give medical words personal nicknames and even know how to select the words you're willing to learn. A keen study into this book has shown you that medical terminologies didn't come from space but are words that originated from Greek and Latin. Additions of prefixes or suffixes will not only give the appropriate meaning to the word root but also give the direction as to how to use them. Don't forget about pluralism when needed. You will agree that even the longest medical term isn't rocket science; you only have to break it down into the word part to examine the individual words. You now have insight into some diagnostic procedures, surgical and medical interventions, and even basic pharmacological terms you'll come across in your practice. Not forgetting some great scientists that have their names after discoveries or inventions, who knows, you could be one too.

As you know that the human body consists of many cells, tissues, organs, and systems that come together and function to maintain life and balance. Realizing how important but easy the systems' terms are, make this book your best friend so that in no time, you will be amazed at how great you've become with simple medical terminologies. Yes! I see greatness in you as you enjoy your medical practice.

APPENDIX
Answers To Quick Exercises

Quick Exercise 1

1. Attention, Interest & Emotions.
2. Recalled.

Quick Exercise 2

1. Personal Nick Name.
2. Scapula = scar +pull +her

Stomach = stole + mark

Nodular = know + do + lah

Ventricle = vent + real +cool

(*other words that sound alike may also be used)*

3. True.

Quick Exercise 3

1. Thalamus.
2. True.
3. Why am I in Med school?

What difference does it make?

Can I do this?

Quick Exercise 4

1. Combining vowels.

2. True.

3. Mediolateral, Pharmacokinetics, Esophagogastroscopy, Cephalocaudal

(other words are also applicable).

4. Menopause = men (word root) o (combining vowel) pause (suffix)

Hemorrhagic = hem (word root) o (combining vowel) rrhagic (suffix)

Cholelithiasis = chol (word root) e (combining vowel) lith (word root) iasis (suffix)

Homeopathy = home (word root) o (combining vowel) pathy (suffix)

Quick Exercise 5

1. Numbers, Colors, Negativity, Direction, Degree, Size and Comparison, Time, Position/Location, Special qualities.
2. Around = (Peri) position/location Large = (Macro) size

Two = (Bi) numbers

Many = (Poly) numbers

All = (Pan) special qualities

Red = (Erythro) color

Death = (Necro) special qualities Away = (Ab) direction

Quick Exercise 6

1. True.
2. The coronal plane describes an imaginary line that cuts the body into two halves, side by side, while the sagittal plane describes an imaginary

line that cuts the body into two halves, forward and backward.

3. Trunk.
4. Anterior and Inferior.

Abdominal and pelvis.

Thoracic and lumbar.

Quick exercise 7

1. Laparoscopy is a surgical procedure using a keyhole incision to assess the abdominopelvic region, while Laparotomy is also a surgical procedure involving a large incision to the abdomen to assess the abdominopelvic region.
2. Light amplification by stimulated emission of radiation.
3. False, it is from a Greek word.
4. Allopurinol, Probenecid.

Quick Exercise 8

1. PTSD = Posttraumatic stress disorder

CAT = Computed axial tomography

TAH = Total abdominal hysterectomy

CBC = Complete blood count

2. APGAR score was discovered by Apgar Virginia in 1953
3. Acetabulum = Acetabula (replacing “um” with “a”)

Appendix = Appendices (replacing “x” with “ces”)

Coccus = Cocci (replacing “us” with “I”)

Quick Exercise 9

1. A.
2. B.
3. Oxygen and carbon dioxide.
4. C.
5. D.
6. To drain blood from the tissues of the heart.

Quick Exercise 10

1. B.
2. A.
3. C.

4. C.
5. Maintenance of Homeostasis.

Memory and learning.

Programming of the spinal cord.

Control of voluntary movement.

6. C.

Quick Exercise 11

7. B.
8. A.
9. 2.
10. Acromegaly.
11. A.
12. A.

Quick Exercise 12

1. A.
2. B.
3. B.
4. Smell, touch, vision, hearing, and taste.

REFERENCES

Anthony Metivier and Jamie Clarke, MD. (2013). How to learn and memorize medical terminology: Using a memory palace specifically designed for achieving medical fluency. (1st ed.). Publisher: Metivier Magnetic Memory Series.

Beverly Henderson, CMT-R, HRT and Jennifer Dorsey, PhD. (2020). Medical terminology for dummies. (3rd ed.), Publisher: John Wiley & Sons, Inc.

Barbara Janson Cohen and MEd Ann DePetris, MSA, RN, CCRP. (2017). Medical terminology: an illustrated guide. (8th ed.). Publisher: Wolters Kluwer.

Bruce Wingerd, (2019). Medical terminology complete. (4th ed.). Publisher: Pearson Education.

Barbara A. Gylys BS, MEd, CMA-A (AAMA) and Regina M. Masters, BSN, MEd, RN, CMA (AAMA). (2014). Medical terminology simplified: A programmed learning approach by body system, (5th ed.). Publisher: Quincy McDonald.

Carolyn Perry MSc, Ph.D. (2021, September 30). Anatomical and medical prefixes and suffixes, Kenhub.com. https://www.kenhub.com/en/library/anatomy/commonly-used-prefixes-in-anatomy.

David Macias, MD. (2021). First MTP joint interposition arthroplasty. Footcaremd. https://www.footcaremd.org/conditions-treatments/toes/first-mtp-joint-interposition-arthroplasty.

Eva Regan. (2016). Medical terminology made easy: Breakdown the language of medicine and quickly build your medical vocabulary. (1st ed.). Publisher: Eva Regan.

Ehlion Team. Medical terminology – Comprehensive list of medical terms. Ehlion.com. https://ehlion.com/magazine/medical-terminology-list/

Jonathan E. Kaplan, MD. (2020, July 28). Antiretrovirals: HIV and AIDS drugs. Webmd.com. https://www.webmd.com/hiv-aids/aids-hiv-medication.

Jasvinder Chawla, MD, MBA. (2018, September 11). Which medications in the drug class, Sedative-Hypnotics, are used in the treatment of Insomnia? Medscape.com. https://www.medscape.com/answers/1187829-75643/which-medications-in-the-drug-class-sedative-hypnotics-are-used-in-the-treatment-of-insomnia.

Johns Hopkins University. (2021). Craniotomy, Hopkinsmedicine-org. https://www-hopkinsmedicine-org.cdn.ampproject.org/v/s/www.hopkinsmedicine.org/health/treatment-tests-and-therapies/craniotomy?amp_js_v=a6&amp_gsa=1&amp=true&usqp=mq331AQKKAFQArABIIACAw%3D%3D#aoh=16343325144602&referrer=https%3A%2F%2Fwww.google.com&amp_tf=From%20%251%24s&ampshare=https%3A%2F%2Fwww.hopkinsmedicine.org%2Fhealth%2Ftreatment-tests-and-therapies%2Fcraniotomy

Jon Johnson. (2020, October 5). Types and side effects of antiemetic drugs. Medicalnewstoday. https://www.medicalnewstoday.com/articles/320384.

Kavitha Ganesan; Muhammad Burhan Majeed Rana; Senan Sultan. (2021, May 15). Oral Hypoglycemic medications. National Centre for Biotechnology Information, https://www.ncbi.nlm.nih.gov/books/NBK482386/

Macmillan Dictionary. (2021). Words used to describe medical treatments, appliances and medicines. Macmillandictionary.com. https://www.macmillandictionary.com/thesaurus-category/british/words-used-to-describe-medical-treatments-appliances-and-medicines.

Meditec. Forming plurals of medical words. Meditec.com. https://www.meditec.com/resourcestools/medical-words/medical-plurals.

Mike Cadogan. (2020, December 18). Cheyne-Stokes respiration, Litfl.com. https://litfl.com/cheyne-stokes-respiration-eponymictionary/

Pharmapproach. (2021, February 22). Common prefixes, roots and suffixes in medical terminology. Pharmapproach.com, https://www.pharmapproach.com/common-prefixes-roots-and-suffixes-in-medical-terminology/

Randall A. Simmons, M.Ed., CRCR, (2019). Medical terminology quick learn. (1st ed.), Publisher: Quick learn guides.

Stephanie Watson. (2018, September 27). Uvula removal surgery. Healthline. https://www.healthline.com/health/uvula-removal.

Wolters Kluwer, Lippincot Williams and Wilkins. (2009). Medical terminology made incredibly easy (3rd ed.). Publisher: Judith A. Schilling McCann, RN, MSN

www.ingramcontent.com/pod-product-compliance
Lightning Source LLC
LaVergne TN
LVHW052302200926
848481LV00002B/436